STRUCTURED EXERCISES in WELLNESS PROMOTION

A WHOLE PERSON™ HANDBOOK FOR TRAINERS, EDUCATORS AND GROUP LEADERS

VOLUME II

edited by
Nancy Loving Tubesing, EdD
and
Donald A Tubesing, MDiv, PhD

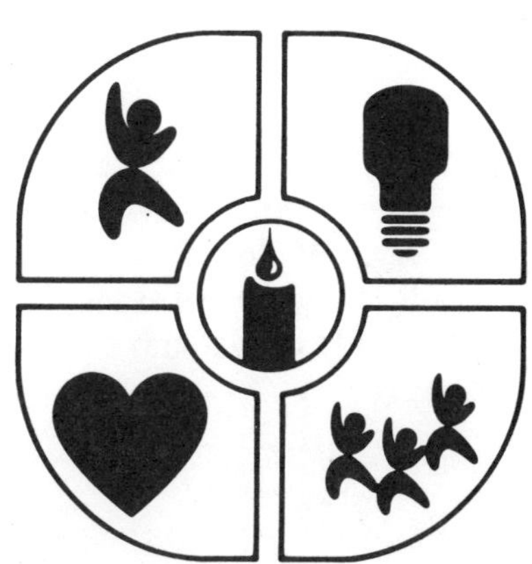

Whole Person Press

Library of Congress Catalog Card Number:
ISBN: 0-938586-04-1

Printed in the United States of America by Port Cities Printing, Superior WI

10 9 8 7 6 5 4 3 2

Published by: **WHOLE PERSON PRESS**
PO Box 3151
Duluth MN 55803
218/728-4077

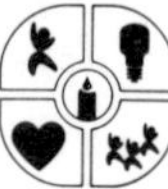

PREFACE

Two years ago we launched an experiment in health education -- The Whole Person Handbook series of Structured Exercises in Stress Management and Wellness Promotion. We believed then that the time had come to move beyond peptalks and handouts to an experiential approach that actively involves the participant -- as a whole person -- in the learning process.

The experiment has been an enormous success! The handbooks have found their way into the libraries of trainers, consultants, counselors, teachers, pastors, adult educators, nurses, managers, group workers, health educators, chaplains, psychologists and physicians around the world. We're proud that these Volumes have been a catalyst for dramatic changes in health education.

Volumes II of the Whole Person Handbooks in Stress and Wellness carry on the tradition of excellence started by their predecessors. Each Handbook contains 36 new structured exercises, complete with step by step instructions for easy use. Some utilize new applications of familiar group processes and techniques. Others were submitted by people like you who continually strive to add the creative touch in their teaching. All have been field-tested with a variety of audiences.

Please note our policy for reproduction of the Handbook contents. Our purpose in publishing these volumes is to foster interprofessional networking and to provide a framework through which we can all share our most effective ideas with each other. The layout is designed for easy photocopying of worksheets and training notes.

Feel free to adapt and duplicate any sections of the Handbook for your use in training or educational events -- as long as you use the proper citation as indicated on the facing page. However, all materials are still covered by copyright. Prior written permission from Whole Person Press is required if you plan large-scale reproduction or distribution of any portion of the Handbook. If you wish to include any material in another publication for sale, please send us your request and proposal.

In the Whole Person Handbook series we've shared our best with you and hope you'll return the favor. We encourage you to submit your favorite structured exercises for inclusion in future volumes. You'll find instructions in the contributor's section at the back of the book. Let us know what works well for you so that we can carry on the tradition of providing a forum for the exchange of innovative teaching designs.

Duluth MN
October 1984

Nancy Loving Tubesing
Donald A Tubesing

WHOLE PERSON ASSOCIATES INC
consultants and publishers

specialists in stress and wellness
programs with a whole person focus

CONSULTATION

- + development and implementation of stress management and wellness programs for clients around the world
- + curriculum design
- + creative problem solving
- + interdisciplinary think tank

CONTINUING EDUCATION

- + workshops, inservice training, keynote speeches, conferences on stress, burnout, wellness, self-care, vitality, communication
- + for professional organizations, community-based helping agencies, hospitals, business, government, education, civic groups

PRODUCT DEVELOPMENT

- + research and development of wellness-oriented products for health-conscious businesses and institutions
- + design of creative stress management premiums and promotions for employees, clients, customers

PUBLISHING

- + Stress and Wellness Handbook series for trainers, educators and group leaders
- + innovative training materials, tape and workbook packages
- + unique "workshop-in-a-book" self-help guides
- + practical "workshop-in-a-box" cassette tape programs
- + unusual relaxation tapes
- + health-related educational games

TABLE OF CONTENTS

ICEBREAKERS

WELLNESS EXPLORATION

SELF-CARE STRATEGIES

ACTION PLANNING / CLOSURE

GROUP ENERGIZERS

INTRODUCTION

Wellness is the hot topic of the 80's. If you're prepared to address the issue, you'll get plenty of opportunities. If you creatively involve people in the learning process, your teaching will be much more helpful than even the most entertaining lecture.

Effective teaching helps people move beyond information to implementation. Health education that really works involves people in the process of reflecting, assessing, prioritizing, sorting, planning for change and affirming progress.

Structured Exercises in Wellness Promotion Volume II offers you 36 designs you can use for getting people involved, whatever the setting and time constraints, whatever the sophistication of the audience. To aid you in the selection of appropriate exercises, they are grouped into five broad categories:

Icebreakers: These short (10-20 minutes) exercises are designed to introduce people to each other and to open up participants' thinking process regarding wellness. They are lively. All seven engage people actively in the topic and with each other. Try combining an icebreaker with an exercise from the wellness or self-care section for an instant evening program.

Wellness Exploration: These exercises explore the issue of wellness from the whole person perspective. Rather than focus merely on the physical, these five processes help people examine their overall lifestyle. You'll find a mixture of moderate length assessments (30-60 minutes) and major theme developers (60-120 minutes). Each exercise can easily be contracted or expanded to fit your purpose.

Self-Care Strategies: The first two exercises help participants examine their self-care goals. The next eight focus on specific self-care strategies in six life dimensions: physical, emotional, mental, spiritual, relational and lifestyle well-being. The last exercise promotes personal responsibility for self-care.

Action Planning/Closure: These five exercises help participants draw together their insights and determine the actions they wish to take on their own behalf. Some of the activities also suggest rituals that bring closure to the group process.

Energizers: The ten energizers are designed to perk up the group whenever fatigue sets in. Sprinkle them throughout your program as needed for a change of pace. Try one as an icebreaker. They're guaranteed to get everyone's juices (including yours!) flowing again in 5-10 minutes.

The Handbook format is designed for easy use. You'll find that each exercise is described completely, including;

- goals
- group size
- time frame
- materials needed
- step-by-step process instructions
- variations

Special instructions to the trainer are typed in italics.
Scripts to be read to the group are typed in a sans serif face.
Questions to ask the group are preceded by a □.
Mini-lecture notes are preceded by a ● or a *.

The instructions are written primarily for large group (30-100 people) workshop settings, but most of the exercises work just as well with small groups, in individual therapy and for personal reflection.

If you are teaching in the workshop or large group setting, we believe that the use of small discussion groups is the most potent learning structure available to you. We've found that groups of four persons each provide ample "air time" and a good variety of interaction. Let groups meet together two or three different times before forming new groups.

These personal "sharing groups" allow people to make positive contact with each other and encourage them to personalize their experience in depth. On evaluations, some people will say, "drop this," others will say, "give us more small group time," but most will report that the time you give them to share with each other becomes the heart of the workshop.

If you are working with an intact group of 12 people or less, you may at times want to keep the whole group together for process and discussion time rather than divide into the suggested four or six person groups.

Each trainer has personal strengths, biases, pet concepts and processes. We expect and encourage you to expand and modify what you find here to accommodate your style. Adjust the exercises as you see fit. Bring these designs to life for your participants by inserting your own content and examples into your teaching. Experiment!

And when you come up with something new, let us know . . .

ICEBREAKERS

37 INTRODUCTIONS 3 (p 1)

In these three get-acquainted exercises participants articulate their expectations (ROUNDUP), affirm their uniqueness (DIFFERENCES) and use an object close at hand to introduce themselves (POCKET OR PURSE).

38 "QUALITY" CIRCLES (p 4)

Participants choose one characteristic of whole person well-being to wear on their name tags. They then use that "quality" to introduce themselves in the circle.

39 ATTENTION TO TENSION (p 6)

In this ice breaker participants identify personal tension patterns and in small groups brainstorm tension-reduction techniques.

40 SILENT AUCTION (p 8)

Participants bid on wellness goals using as currency action steps they know would help them reach the goal(s). This exercise in creativity and commitment works well as an icebreaker, closing planner or health fair activity.

41 VITALITY SCORE (p 14)

This introductory exercise quickly engages participants in a consideration of the broad view of wellness as overall vitality and personal energy. It can be used effectively as an energizer in a short speech or as part of a longer workshop.

37 INTRODUCTIONS 3

In these three get-acquainted exercises participants articulate their expectations (ROUNDUP), affirm their uniqueness (DIFFERENCES) and use an object close at hand to introduce themselves (POCKET OR PURSE).

GOALS

1) To promote interaction and help participants get acquainted.

2) To focus the group's attention on one aspect of the topic of wellness.

GROUP SIZE

Unlimited; modifications may be required for large groups as noted below.

TIME FRAME

10-15 minutes or longer, depending on the size of the group

PROCESS

ROUNDUP

Note: This process is most effective when paired with the closing exercise, ROUNDUP REVISITED, p 98.

1) The trainer points out that everyone has come to this session with her own unique set of expectations. He gives a few examples such as, "I hope to get motivated about daily exercise" or "I hope to meet some people with similar interests."

2) Participants are invited to silently review their expectations and choose one to share with the group.

3) Beginning with the trainer, each person briefly (30 seconds or less) completes the sentence:
   * "My name is _______ and my expectation for today's workshop/class/session is _______."

   Note: Do not ask for explanations or permit comments. Do allow people to "pass".

4) The trainer summarizes what he has heard, noting that some of the expectations expressed may be met completely,

others not at all. He encourages participants to take responsibility for getting their own needs met, suggesting alternative resources where appropriate. This is a good time for the trainer to outline his agenda for the meeting.

VARIATIONS

- Alternative sentences that could be used in the ROUNDUP:
  - "My personal goal for this session is . . ."
  - "One thing I can contribute to this workshop is . ."

DIFFERENCES

1) Participants are asked to look around the group and identify several ways they are different from everyone else in the group.

2) One by one participants introduce themselves, stating their name and one characteristic that makes them unique. Each person must choose a different "difference".

   Note: The trainer may want to give an example such as, "I'm (name) and one way I imagine I'm different is that my grandfather was a Sioux Indian." Or, "I'm (name) and I'm the tallest person here."

VARIATIONS

- If the group is larger than 15-20 people, it may take more than 15 minutes to complete this exercise. However, the larger the number of participants, the more challenging will be the learning experience as participants struggle to find "new" ways to be "different"!

  Depending on the group size and the time available, the trainer may choose to divide participants into smaller groups (6-10 people) for this exercise.

- Introductions could be expanded to include similarities as well as differences. Participants identify one way they are similar to others in the group and use this as well as their unique quality in introducing themselves.

POCKET OR PURSE

1) The trainer asks participants to find something in their pocket or purse, or to choose something they are wearing, that symbolizes their current state of health or one of their health concerns.

2) Participants introduce themselves to the group, showing their symbolic object and describing how it relates to their current health status.

   Note: The trainer may want to share first as a model. (eg "I'm (name) and I choose these earrings which were my grandmother's. She lived alone and was still taking courses at the U when she died at 93. I expect to live that long and stay just as lively." Or, I"m (name) and I picked this aspirin bottle -- I've got arthritis real bad and need to learn new ways to deal with my pain.")

VARIATIONS

- In a large group (more than 20 people), the trainer may want to divide participants into sharing units of 4-12 people for these introductions.

ROUNDUP is a modification of Sid Simon's "Values Whip" introduced to us by Lois Hart.

38 "QUALITY" CIRCLES

Participants choose one characteristic of whole person well-being to wear on their name tags. They then use that "quality" to introduce themselves in the circle.

GOALS

1) To highlight the whole person nature of health.

2) To promote interaction and help people get acquainted.

GROUP SIZE

Unlimited

TIME FRAME

10-15 minutes

MATERIALS NEEDED

1½" X 2" yellow POST-IT notes (available at office supply stores).

PROCESS

Note: Before the meeting, the trainer needs to prepare health "quality" stickers. Use POST-IT notes, writing one attribute from the list below on each separate sticker, then posting them all on the wall, blackboard or newsprint where participants can have easy access. Make plenty of stickers so that the last people still have some choices. Feel free to make up additional qualities if more are needed.

1) As participants arrive for the session, they are asked to choose one health "quality" sticker from those posted. They attach the POST-IT they have selected to their name tag.

2) When everyone is present, the trainer designates five areas in the room where groups can gather, naming them "physical", "emotional", "mental", "interpersonal" and "spiritual" health. Participants are asked to look at their health quality POST-IT, decide which dimension of well-being it best represents and move to the corresponding area of the room.

   Note: There are no absolutely "right" classifications.

Encourage people to choose the category that makes most sense to them. Don't worry if the groupings that result are uneven in number. The smaller groups can use the extra time to share at more depth or to talk about why so few people chose qualities in their area.

3) Once the groups have gathered in their respective spots, the trainer instructs participants to introduce themselves to their "quality" circle, telling:

   * Name
   * Quality I picked
   * Why I chose this quality
   * How it ties into my overall health

HEALTH QUALITIES

Physical:	strong, energetic, rested, relaxed, tip top shape, self-disciplined, pain-free, athletic, sexy, vital
Mental:	alert, creative, logical, poetic, open-minded, curious, enthusiastic, capable, thoughtful, problem-solver
Emotional:	expressive, stable, self-confident, independent, content, in touch, sensitive, secure, self-aware
Interpersonal:	out-going, honest, tolerant, assertive, helpful, forgiving, affectionate, responsive, caring, respectful
Spiritual:	hopeful, committed, purposeful, trusting, at peace, forgiven, reflective, generous, compassionate, faithful, socially concerned

TRAINER'S NOTES

39 ATTENTION TO TENSION

In this get-acquainted exercise participants identify personal tension patterns and in small groups brainstorm tension-reduction techniques.

GOALS

1) To heighten awareness of physical tension.

2) To explore whole body tension-reduction strategies.

3) To promote interaction and exchange of expertise among participants.

GROUP SIZE

Can be adapted to suit most groups.

TIME FRAME

15-20 minutes

PROCESS

1) The trainer briefly describes the role of tension in overall health and well-being. (5 minutes)

- Most people store leftover tension from stressful situations somewhere in their bodies -- in the back, in the toes, in the chest, in the jaw. No part of the body is immune from potential tension build-up.

- This tension is imperceptible at first, accumulating slowly over the day or week or month until finally we notice its presence in the form of a stiff neck or a headache or a queasy stomach.

- Unless we learn how to interrupt this cycle and to discharge, release or relax this tension, we are putting unnecessary wear and tear on our bodies that may eventually lead to serious health problems.

- The first step toward alleviating this tension is to pay attention to it. Only then can we recognize its presence and take steps to release it.

- The second step is to learn, practice and regularly use specific techniques for letting go of tension in different areas of the body.

2) The trainer indicates that during this exercise participants will attend to their tension, practice relaxation and get acquainted, too!

3) Participants are instructed to close their eyes and mentally scan their bodies from head to toe, noticing any tension spots. (2-3 minutes)

   Note: The trainer may want to be more directive here, instructing the group to take it slowly and guiding the process (head . . . face . . . neck . . . shoulders . . . arms . . . etc, down to toes). A gentle stretch may also increase awareness of tension.

4) After this brief tension check, the trainer asks people to focus on one particular place they found tension during the body scan. Participants are instructed to place one hand on that tension spot.

   As soon as everyone is touching a "hot" spot, the trainer directs them to stand up and move around the room -- still holding their tension area. As soon as they find two other people who are holding the same spot, they are to sit down together and introduce themselves.

5) Once everyone has found a group of three, the trainer invites the trios to continue getting acquainted by describing some of the activities they find useful for relaxing tension in their particular trouble area. When practical, group members may try each technique as it is suggested. (5 minutes)

6) The trainer reconvenes the large group and asks for comments and observations, prompting discussion as necessary with questions like:

   - ☐ Where did most people hold tension?
   - ☐ What were the most common tension-relaxing techniques?
   - ☐ What were some unique techniques for various body areas?
   - ☐ Were there any tension-relievers that would be useful right now? If so, try them with the whole group.

VARIATION

- Instead of the brief tension check in Step 3, the more intensive Body Scanning Exercise, p 113, could be used to help people become more aware of their tension spots.

40 SILENT AUCTION

Participants bid on wellness goals using as currency action steps they know would help them reach the goal(s). This exercise in creativity and commitment works well as an ice-breaker, closing planner, or health fair activity.

GOALS

1) To explore and clarify wellness goals.

2) To activate participants' internal wisdom in identifying action steps for reaching goals.

3) To set a relaxed and playful tone.

GROUP SIZE

Most effective with 8-24 people.

TIME FRAME

20-30 minutes

MATERIALS NEEDED

Roll of blank tickets like those used for carnivals and raffles (available at office supply stores); collection of objects that symbolize wellness goals; "Bidding Forms" for all participants.

PROCESS

Note: Before the session the trainer needs to choose several wellness goals that are appropriate to the group and the course content to be emphasized. For each goal, you will need an object that symbolizes it for the auction (see p 11 for suggestions) and an envelope with the goal written on the outside to be used for receiving bids. Choose many objects for the auction if you wish to stimulate participants to consider several potential areas for change. Limit the items to just a few if you want to help people set priorities and tackle one goal at a time.

When the meeting space is set up, the objects to be auctioned should be arranged on the table so all participants can see them. Put the envelopes next to their symbolic objects. To heighten the suspense, cover the display table with a sheet until Step 5.

1) The trainer introduces the topic of wellness and invites participants to reflect on their personal wellness goals, covering one or more of the following points:

- Within the group there will be diverse as well as common hopes, dreams and expectations. Each of us brings our unique health history and personal agenda to this meeting.

- Goal-setting is an essential ingredient in wellness promotion. Unless we know where we want to go, and what our priorities are, we can't take the necessary steps toward being well.

- Some of us are overwhelmed by the sheer number of goals we could and should be aiming for. Others are immobilized by the enormity of a single goal -- like giving up cigarettes or losing 50 pounds.

- The only way to reach a goal is to decide that it is a priority and then take one small step at a time toward achieving it.

- Most of us have nearly all the information we need to make desired changes. We just need to listen to our internal wisdom, take it seriously and then take action. The issue is commitment and motivation -- we need to put our money where our mouth is!

2) The trainer distributes an equal number of tickets to all participants (10-12 works well), asking everyone to write her name on each of her tickets. These tickets will be used as "currency" for the auction.

3) The trainer describes the silent auction as a playful yet serious way to clarify wellness priorities and to identify specific steps for reaching them. Each participant receives a "Bidding Form" while the trainer gives and demonstrates instructions for the general auction process, using the script below:

There are several objects on this table that represent wellness goals you may wish to achieve. When I remove this cover, you are invited to look over the items to be auctioned and decide which goal or goals you would like to bid on.

Note: The trainer may want to choose one auction item to use as an example during this explanation.

You may bid on as many objects as you wish, using the tickets you received earlier. Each ticket used for a bid must have written on it one action step you could take toward reaching that goal. If you bid five tickets on one goal, you need to write five different action steps.

Bids are made by placing one or more tickets -- complete with action step(s) -- into the envelope representing your desired wellness goal. The winning bid for each goal is determined by who wagers the most (places the most tickets in the corresponding envelope). In case of ties, the winner will be selected by a drawing.

4) The trainer reviews the detailed instructions at the bottom of the "Bidding Form", reminding participants to write their proposed action steps both on the ticket and on the form. The "Bidding Form" thus becomes the participant's personal record of her ideas and commitments.

5) The auction is declared open for bids. If the objects have been hidden, the cover is lifted. The trainer identifies each wellness goal by its symbol and encourages people to gather around the table and take a close look at the items before placing their bids.

6) Participants decide on goals, fill out their tickets and "Bidding Forms" and make their bids by placing their action step tickets in the appropriate envelopes.

   Note: The trainer may want to set a time limit of 5 minutes for the actual bidding. At the end of that time, the envelopes are sealed.

7) The silent part of the auction is now complete and the noise begins. The trainer chooses the envelope and the object representing one of the wellness goals. Participants are asked to shout out their bids for this goal (the number of tickets they deposited in that envelope).

8) The "winner" is asked to come forward, open the envelope and read to the group, one at a time, all the action steps that bidders suggested for reaching this goal. The trainer encourages participants who bid on this goal to jot down the good ideas others have proposed.

9) When all the action steps have been read, the trainer awards the wellness goal symbol as a "treasure" to the highest bidder.

10) Steps 7, 8 and 9 are repeated until all goals have been auctioned.

11) After the auction has been completed the trainer asks for comments, observations and insights from the group.

- ☐ Which goal got the most action? Which little?
- ☐ What does this suggest about the group's priorities? Strengths? Neglected possibilities?
- ☐ What steps are appropriate for reaching <u>any</u> goal?

VARIATION

- Instead of auctioning wellness goals, the group could bid on different topics to be covered during the course or workshop. Limit tickets to three per person and replace the "action steps" with "reasons to study this topic".

WELLNESS GOAL	SYMBOLIC OBJECT
take better care of myself	mirror
live a long life	social security card
lose 10 pounds	calorie chart
lose 30 pounds	Weight Watcher's TV dinner box
lose 50 or more pounds	calorie chart and jumprope
reach my ideal weight	tape measure
regular aerobic exercise	shoe laces
physical fitness	fitness magazine
cut down on smoking	cigarettes with 2-3" cut off
become a non-smoker	empty ash tray
cut down on alcohol	half an aluminum beer can
stop alcohol	Perrier water and car keys
get high on life, not chemicals	Life magazine
reduce salt intake	empty salt shaker, salt substitute
reduce refined sugars	artificial sweetener, fresh fruit
eat well-balanced diet	food from each of "basic four"
fewer empty calories	empty candy bar wrapper
avoid heart attack/cancer	Prevention magazine
figure out what's wrong with me	thermometer
learn how to relax	rubber band
regular, refreshing sleep	pillow
freedom from pain	empty aspirin bottle
to feel better	toy top
to have more energy	battery
to slow down my pace	flower ("smell the flowers")
to raise healthier kids	apple
to grow as a person	seeds
to be kind and caring	warm "fuzzy"
to make friends	HELLO, my name is . . . nametag
to stay lively and creative	light bulb
to be loving and tender	valentine card
to be more flexible	spring from ballpoint pen
hope	cross
relief from depression	cartoon, smiley face sticker
relief from anxiety	"easy does it!" bumper sticker
positive self-image	ID card
peace of mind	candle
forgiveness	rosary

SILENT AUCTION BIDDING FORM

SYMBOL	WELLNESS GOAL	MY BID (one action step for each ticket)
		1) 2) 3)

BIDDING INSTRUCTIONS

You may use one or more tickets to bid on a wellness goal. Before you start, make sure that your name is on one side of the ticket. Think about how many goals you want to bid on and how many tickets you are willing to spend for each. You could bid all your tickets on one very important goal, or bid a few tickets on several goals. You decide.

A. Decide on the first wellness goal you want to bid on.

B. Write the symbol and goal on your Bidding Form (above).

C. Decide how many of your tickets you are willing to risk on this goal. For each ticket, write one action step you could take that would help you reach this goal. Remember, for a valid bid, each action step must be different. Be as specific and creative as possible.

D. Before making your bid, record these action steps from each ticket on your Bidding Form (above).

E. Make your "bid" by putting your tickets in the envelope marked with your wellness goal.

F. If you have any tickets remaining, go back to Step A, decide on another wellness goal and repeat this process, continuing to bid on new goals as long as you have tickets.

41 VITALITY SCORE

This introductory exercise quickly engages participants in a consideration of the broad view of wellness as overall vitality and personal energy. It can be used effectively as an energizer in a short speech or as part of a longer workshop.

GOALS

1) To allow participants an initial contact with each other.

2) To stimulate participants' awareness of their current level of wellness and identification of their vitality level.

GROUP SIZE

Unlimited, works well in large groups and small.

TIME FRAME

5-10 minutes

PROCESS

1) The trainer asks participants each to rate their current wellness/vitality level on a 1-10 scale and to record their personal number in writing.

   Note: *The trainer may point out that a self-rating of "1" would be akin to saying, "I'm so sick I couldn't have gotten here on my own. Four friends must have lowered me in through the ceiling by ropes." A self-rating of "10" would be like saying, "I'm so high and energetic I can hardly stay in this chair." Most, of course, will rate themselves somewhere in between.*

   If some want to know exactly what criteria they should use to determine their rating, simply say, "Base it on your overall energy and vitality level right now."

2) To gather a sense of the group, the trainer asks for a show of hands to the following questions:

   - How many are at a number of "4" or below?
   - How many are at "5", "6", or "7"?
   - How many are at "8" or above?

Note: The trainer may facetiously comment to the "4" and below group, "I know there are more of you out there, but you either didn't hear the question or you simply didn't have the energy to get your hand in the air. We'll try to get you some help today."

To the "8" and above group the trainer may say, "No matter what happens in this seminar, you'll get something out of this day. Some days are like that; you're so high, you'll have a great day no matter what!"

3) The trainer asks participants to jot notes in response to the following sequence of questions:

Note: Encourage participants to write down the first response that crosses their mind.

- □ "At what number would you like your energy level to be today?"
- □ "What number would you like to see in those you live with?"

  Note: The trainer may point out that not everyone wants to live at the "10" level all the time. Certainly most would be irritated by living with someone who's always at "10".

- □ "If you keep living the same way you've lived in the past month, what number do you expect you'll be experiencing one year from today?"

  Note: The trainer may want to pick a date with specific relevance to the group. For example, at a teachers' inservice in October, the question might be, "If you don't change anything, at what number do you expect your energy level will be by next June?"

4) The trainer then invites participants to complete these two sentence stems:

- □ "If I want to move up one number on the vitality scale, I'll probably need to stop ____________."
- □ "If I want to move up one number on the vitality scale, I'll probably need to start ____________."

5) The trainer asks participants to pair up and share their answers to the questions.

6) The trainer reconvenes the group and asks for observations regarding personal vitality and how it is affected by one's lifestyle decisions.

VARIATION

- This sequence of questions could also be used in the Two Minute Mill process, WELLNESS I, p 5.

TRAINER'S NOTES

WELLNESS EXPLORATION

42 INVESTING IN HEALTH (p 17)

This simple health habit assessment compares daily health behaviors with investments in a pension plan, and challenges participants to assess the quantity and quality of the investments they are currently making in their "future health" portfolio.

43 MY PRESENT HEALTH STATUS (p 22)

This exercise allows participants to rank their level of health in a variety of areas, affirming positive behaviors and identifying needed changes.

44 CARING APPRAISAL (p 26)

In this whole health assessment, participants analyze the quality of their self-care habits (body, mind, spirit, relationships) as well as their other-care commitments (family, spouse, neighbors, creation).

45 SICKNESS BENEFITS (p 35)

Participants use a seven-step process to track down the "benefits" they may get from their sickness or its symptoms. They then identify more responsible alternatives for getting their needs met.

46 WHEEL OF HEALTH (p 39)

This extended process helps participants explore the concept of wholeness by involving them in the building of a whole person model and examining the implications of their design. The process includes 3 parts: A) building the wheel model; B) exploring the implications of the wheel; C) self-examination.

42 INVESTING IN HEALTH

This simple health habit assessment compares daily health behaviors with investments in a pension plan, and challenges participants to assess the quantity and quality of the investments they are currently making in their "future health" portfolio.

GOALS

1) To teach participants the "seven basic rules" of health.

2) To demonstrate that future health is the result of current daily health habits.

3) To stimulate healthier choice-making throughout the day.

GROUP SIZE

Unlimited, also effective in work with individuals.

TIME FRAME

10-15 minutes

MATERIALS NEEDED

One copy of the "Health Habit Inventory" and "Today's Investment Decisions" for each participant.

PROCESS

1) The trainer introduces the exercise by outlining the following chalk talk concepts:

   - Faulty living patterns take their toll on future health. Every major degenerative disease due to stress-full living is predictable and preventable in its first decade of development. Disease takes a long time to develop. Numerous signs and symptoms, warnings that something is wrong, appear long before a disease can be officially named. Stress-related diseases due to long term investment in a faulty lifestyle are not chance occurrences. They are self-made; the results are self-imposed.

   - Health is a return on investment. Maximum long-term health is most likely to be found in individuals who choose to invest their energies in a health-enhancing lifestyle. Health-producing habits are the world's best medicine.

- <u>You become your investments</u>. Most people regularly pay into a pension plan designed to provide financial security in retirement years. The amount that is put into the plan each day is very small, but over the years it adds up.

  Everyone builds a health pension plan, too. The long-range investments we make in our health accumulate over the years. Viewed on a day-to-day basis, our investment in a nap after lunch, a phone call to a friend, or a five-minute break to watch the sunset doesn't seem to have much long-term effect on our health. That extra cup of coffee, one more rushed hour, another angry agrument, or a cynical remark don't seem as if they should detract from our health 20 years from now. But they do. These little bits do add up over the long run.

- <u>We alone make our investment decisions</u>. Remember, to a large extent we are in control of how we look and feel 10, 20, 30 years from now. We're in the process of determining that future today. Let's take the mystery out of lifestyle-related disease. We earn it. We harvest what we sow. We get what we deserve.

  We don't have to change if we don't want to. We can go ahead and continue the habits we want to keep. Only it is important that we know what we're investing in. Is it a long term investment in health or dis-ease? What's the price, what's the reward, of continuing more of the same? We decide!

2) Participants complete the seven question "Health Habit Inventory".

3) The trainer gives background information on the origin of this inventory:

   - These seven true-false questions were used in a massive study in Alameda County, California, conducted by the UCLA School of Public Health. Researchers collected data on thousands of residents, then analyzed it, searching for clues regarding the long term effect of these health behaviors.

   - The mortality table on the worksheet compares the reported death rate by age categories of those who practice 6 or 7 of these health habits, with those who practice 0-3 health habits.

4) The trainer asks for reactions and comments from the group regarding the reported death rates. The trainer may ask, "What is the message in this data?" (One joker responded, "The moral is, 'live like hell until you're 54 and then shape up'")

5) The trainer asks participants to complete the worksheet portion entitled, "Today's Investment Decisions".

6) Again, as before, comments may be solicited from the group.

VARIATIONS

- Following Step 5, participants may be divided into small groups and asked to share their answers and their insights.

TRAINER'S NOTES

HEALTH HABIT INVENTORY

Mark each statement either True or False

T F 1) I don't smoke cigarettes.

T F 2) I do not down more than four alcoholic drinks at a stretch.

T F 3) I regularly eat breakfast.

T F 4) I don't eat between meals.

T F 5) I maintain normal weight.

T F 6) I sleep seven or eight hours a day.

T F 7) I exercise moderately.

MORTALITY TABLE

Following are the death rates over a 5½ year period of two groups of men and women identified in some Alameda studies:

Death Rate of Those Maintaining 6-7 Good Health Habits	Age Group	Death Rate of Those Maintaining 0-3 Good Health Habits
1 percent	Under 45	2 percent
4 percent	45-54	5 percent
6 percent	55-64	17 percent
11 percent	65-74	38 percent
13 percent	Over 75	69 percent

TODAY'S INVESTMENT DECISIONS

What little favors have you done for yourself today that will add up to long-range investments in your health. (Examples: leisurely balanced breakfast, walk to work, affirming phone call, three deep breaths)

Multiplied 10,000 times over the next 30 years, these activities will help immensely in moving you toward your health-investment goals.

Now the other side of the balance sheet. What insults have you offered yourself today that are long-range investments in a future disabling illness? (Examples: three cups of coffee, rushing to meet the bus, shouting at the kids, beer and popcorn at the game)

Multiplied 10,000 times over the next 30 years, these and other negative self-care habits will probably kill you!

Are there any changes you would like to make?

43 MY PRESENT HEALTH STATUS

This exercise allows participants to rank their level of health in a variety of areas, affirming positive behaviors and identifying needed changes.

GOALS

1) To raise participants' consciousness about the many dimensions of health.

2) To assess well-being in a variety of areas.

GROUP SIZE

Unlimited, as long as there is space for groups of four to spread themselves throughout the room.

TIME REQUIRED

30-40 minutes

MATERIALS NEEDED

"My Present Health Status" worksheets.

PROCESS

1) The trainer introduces the concept of health status and the variety of ways that people can measure their well-being.

2) The trainer distributes "My Present Health Status" worksheets to all participants.

3) Beginning with the section labelled "Exercise," the trainer asks participants to reflect on the healthfulness of their current patterns and then to mark their exercise "health status" on the line somewhere between 0 and 7 (0 = abysmal, 7 = outstanding).

   As they consider where to place themselves, participants should write in the box to the left of the "0" all those habits, activities and attitudes which would influence them to judge their exercise status as less healthy. In the box to the right of "7," participants can list all those behaviors and attitudes that contribute in a positive way to their exercise health status.

Once people have marked their status and recorded the influencing factors, the trainer asks them to note any observations that strike them about this area of health.

4) The trainer continues to guide participants through the worksheet, one section at a time, using the same process as outlined in Step 3.

5) When the entire worksheet is completed, the trainer may ask participants to turn the sheet over and write a summary of their health status, as if it were to be included in a medical chart. The summary could include:
   * brief statement of health problems
   * list of specific changes that would enhance their well-being
   * list of personal health resources and accomplishments

6) The trainer asks participants to divide themselves into groups of 4 and find a spot in the room that gives them some privacy. Once everyone has settled down, the trainer asks people to read their summaries to the others in their group and to discuss their observations.

VARIATIONS

- Instead of writing a health status summary (Step 5), participants could write a letter to themselves from their "personal health consultant" who would highlight "well dones" and point out areas where there's "room for improvement."

- Following Step 4 or Step 5, the trainer could ask participants to reflect on what they have discovered and to jot down their first responses to the following sentence stems . . .
   * I am most proud of . . .
   * I am most worried about . . .
   * I don't care about . . .
   * I'd better do something about . . .
   * There's no point in . . .
   * I'm most surprised . . .

- Step 5 may be dropped. Participants move directly from the health status rankings to sharing in small groups.

TRAINER'S NOTES

MY PRESENT HEALTH STATUS

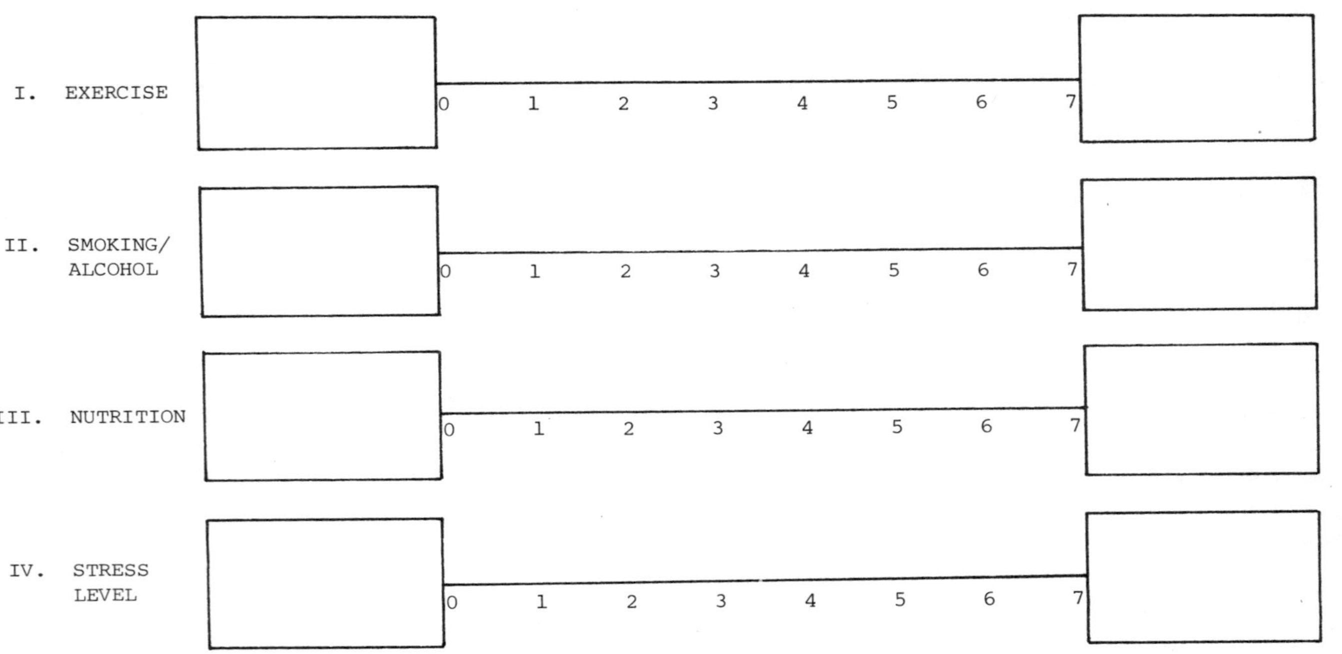

V. SPIRIT		0	1	2	3	4	5	6	7	
VI. RELATION-SHIPS INTIMACY/ SUPPORT		0	1	2	3	4	5	6	7	
VII. LIFE WORK		0	1	2	3	4	5	6	7	
VIII. ENERGY LEVEL		0	1	2	3	4	5	6	7	
IX. OVERALL HEALTH		0	1	2	3	4	5	6	7	

44 CARING APPRAISAL

In this whole health assessment, participants analyze the quality of their self-care habits (body, mind, spirit, relationships) as well as their other-care commitments (family, spouse, neighbors, creation).

GOALS

1) To help participants assess their self-care habits--body, mind, spirit and relationships.

2) To encourage participants to see that the "truly well" care for others, too!

GROUP SIZE

Unlimited, also effective with individuals.

TIME FRAME

45-60 minutes

MATERIALS NEEDED

One copy of the "Health Habit Inventory" and "Caring Question Outreach Appraisal" for each participant.

PROCESS

1) The trainer introduces this appraisal by outlining the following concepts:

   - Health and wellness are more than simply "having a body that works". Well beings exhibit functioning bodies, active minds, clear spirits and loving relationships. One may have a body that's finely tuned and still be sick. Another may be quite well while inhabiting a body that no longer works as it is supposed to. Wellness is a whole-person issue.

   - Self-care health habits in every aspect of life (body, mind, spirit, relationships) may either add to or detract from one's overall well-being. While each is important, seldom do people care for themselves equally in all dimensions.

   - Truly healthy people are "well-to-do . . .". They know that the focus on wellness as an end in itself is too shallow and self-centered. To be fully well, one must do something with that wellness -- one must reach out with care for others to make a positive difference in the world.

2) Participants are instructed to complete the self-care "Health Habit Inventory", answering the questions either "yes" or "no" as accurately as they can. (Admittedly, some answers will be "mostly yes" or "mostly no.") Participants then total their "yes" responses in each category.

3) The trainer helps participants interpret their score by making the following comments:

- Your total of "yes" responses on the Health Habit Inventory provides a general idea of how well you take care of your health across all dimensions of life. Compare your total score to the Caring Question Standards:

24-28	*Excellent:*	*Your habits are enhancing your health.*
16-23	*Average:*	*You're obviously trying, but there's room for improvement.*
Below 16	*Poor:*	*The quality of your health is probably diminished by your poor habits.*

- For specifics on your self-care style, pay particular attention to your score in each of the four categories: physical, mental, relational and spiritual.

- If you recorded three or fewer "yes" responses in any dimension, you're neglecting your health in that area. If you aren't yet experiencing symptoms, you probably soon will. You may wish to take action to modify your habits.

- In those areas where you answered "yes" four or five times, you're probably taking adequate care of yourself. Your self-care habits do enhance your health, but you might consider upgrading your style for optimal health-fullness. There's still room for improvement.

- "Yes" responses to six or seven questions in any category indicates that you are practicing positive self-care habits. Congratulations! Over the long run your choices will enhance the quality of your life and your health.

4) The trainer instructs participants to complete the section entitled, "Personal Reflection on my Self-Care Patterns".

5) Participants are instructed to complete the "Caring Question Outreach Appraisal" answering the questions either "yes" or "no" as before. Participants then total their "yes" responses in each category.

Note: Participants answer either the "For Singles Only" or the "For Marrieds Only" questions, but not both.

6) The trainer helps participants interpret their score by making the following comments:

- Your total of "yes" answers on the Outreach Inventory provides you with an indication of your investments in service and self-sacrifice. Compare your total score with the Caring Question Standards:

21-24	*Excellent:*	*You're obviously intent on making a positive difference in your world.*
12-19	*Average:*	*You do reach out, but you might consider expanding your reach.*
Below 12	*Poor:*	*You're in danger of being self-engrossed.*

- For specifics on your self-sacrifice patterns, pay particular attention to your score in each of the categories. Your answers indicate your priorities. Did you total very few "yes" responses in one category but many in another? Where are your strengths in reaching out? Where are your weaknesses?

- Obviously, you can't reach out everywhere at once. Do your answers adequately reflect your values? Is any adjustment needed? If you recorded three or fewer "yes" responses in any category, you may be neglecting your responsibility to reach out in that area.

7) The trainer instructs participants to complete the section entitled, "Personal Reflections on My Well-To-Do Pattern".

8) The trainer divides participants into groups of four persons each (or utilizes previously established discussion groups). Participants are instructed to spend 4-5 minutes each sharing as much as they like about their self-care and other-care patterns, and their

personal resolutions based on these patterns. After each participant has shared his own profile, the small group may discuss similarities and differences they noticed in the four separate care patterns exhibited by group members. (20-30 minutes)

9) Following the sharing in small groups, the trainer reconvenes the entire group and asks for observations and insights.

The trainer may also ask for a show of hands indicating which areas of wellness are best cared for and which neglected. If this exercise is conducted early in the course, the trainer may want to note areas of particular need exhibited by the group, and plan future teaching segments accordingly.

VARIATIONS

- If time is short, the group discussion time could be cut. However, experience indicates that the discussion time centering on this appraisal is of great value.

TRAINER'S NOTES

The "Health Habit Inventory" and "Caring Question Outreach Appraisal" are excerpted with permission from The Caring Question by Donald A Tubesing and Nancy Loving Tubesing (Minneapolis: Augsburg Publishing House, 1983). This book offers chapter-by-chapter discussion on each of the eight caring dimensions included in the CARING APPRAISAL.

HEALTH HABIT INVENTORY

Yes No

PHYSICAL

____ ____ I participate regularly (three times a week or more) in a vigorous physical exercise program.

____ ____ I eat a well-balanced diet.

____ ____ My weight is within 10 lbs of the ideal weight for my height.

____ ____ My alcohol consumption is seven drinks (shot, beer, or glass of wine) or fewer per week.

____ ____ I always wear my seat belt.

____ ____ I do not smoke cigarettes, cigars or a pipe.

____ ____ I generally get adequate and satisfying sleep.

MENTAL

____ ____ I seldom experience periods of depression.

____ ____ I generally face up to problems and cope with change effectively.

____ ____ I worry very little about future possibilities or things I can't change.

____ ____ I laugh several times a day and usually fit "play" into my schedule.

____ ____ I am curious and always on the lookout for new learning.

____ ____ I maintain a realistic and basically positive self-image.

____ ____ I choose to feel confident and optimistic.

RELATIONAL

____ ____ I seek help and support when I need it.

____ ____ I have at least one friend with whom I can share almost anything.

____ ____ I have nourishing intimate relationships with family and/or friends.

____ ____ I experience and express a wide range of emotions and respond to others' feelings appropriately.

____ ____ Each day includes comfortable and stimulating interaction with others, frequently new acquaintances.

____ ____ I solicit and accept feedback from others.

____ ____ I stick up for myself when it's necessary and appropriate.

Yes	No	
		SPIRITUAL
_____	_____	I set aside 15-20 minutes each day for prayer or meditation.
_____	_____	I participate in regular spiritual rituals with people who share my beliefs.
_____	_____	I accept my limitations and inadequacies without embarrassment or apology.
_____	_____	I keep the purpose of my life clearly in mind and let it guide my goal-setting and decision-making.
_____	_____	I regularly offer my time and possessions in service to others.
_____	_____	I am sensitive to ultimate truths and the spiritual dimension of life.
_____	_____	I readily forgive myself and others.

Count up your "yes" responses for each category and record them below.

Physical	_____	"Yes" responses
Mental	_____	"Yes" responses
Relational	_____	"Yes" responses
Spiritual	_____	"Yes" responses
Total	_____	Out of 28 questions

PERSONAL REFLECTION ON MY SELF-CARE PATTERNS

Please answer these questions on the reverse side or on blank paper.

- □ In which areas are your habits an asset?
- □ In which areas are your habits a liability?
- □ In which areas would you like to make changes?
- □ Which particular habits would you like to modify?

CARING QUESTION OUTREACH APPRAISAL

Yes No

FAMILY

_____ _____ Staying in touch with my extended family is a top priority for me.

_____ _____ I readily accept the responsibility to care for dependent family members who are less able than I because of age, health or abilities.

_____ _____ I hug all members of my family regularly and directly communicate my caring for them in other ways.

_____ _____ I have said "no" to stimulating life options in order to care for my family. For periods of time I have made my family's welfare more important than my own.

_____ _____ I find it possible to accept and affirm each family member as he or she is, complete with strengths and weaknesses, beauty and blemishes.

_____ _____ I regularly participate in family time: special rituals, celebrations and traditions that promote communication and a positive history.

NEIGHBORS

_____ _____ I respect others for their uniqueness and do not find it necessary to try to make them be like me.

_____ _____ I try to personally touch each person I meet each day with kindness and warmth.

_____ _____ I practice being attentive to the needs of others around me--even if they're not spoken. I'm willing to bear others' burdens in any way I can.

_____ _____ I am a good listener and can listen empathically without judgment.

_____ _____ I volunteer to share my gifts for the good of others both in my close neighborhood and beyond.

_____ _____ I tell others what I appreciate about them.

CREATION

_____ _____ I am committed to a cause beyond myself, and I invest some of my money, my time and my energy in it.

_____ _____ I feel compassion for all and I feel pain whenever anyone is put down or held back because of their race, sex or religious views. Whenever I see this occur, I speak up.

_____ _____ I try to consume only what I need and take pride in moving through the world lightly and living simply. My life is not overburdened with "things".

_____ _____ I feel personally responsible to keep the environment clean, often stopping to pick up cans, wrappers, etc.

_____ _____ I have a balanced perspective on the purpose and use of money and do not stack it up for its own sake.

_____ _____ I am determined that because I am here, this world will be a better place to live than it would have been without me.

Note: Complete only one of the next two sections -- whichever applies to you.

Yes	No	
		FOR SINGLES ONLY
_____	_____	I accept myself as a single person and believe that God accepts me and my feelings.
_____	_____	I live in the "now" as a single, free to be me, rather than yearning for a past or future partner.
_____	_____	I am clear about who I am, my purpose in life and my values.
_____	_____	I search for intimacy in the context of my personal guidelines for responsible sexuality.
_____	_____	I am assertive about filling my calendar and my life with meaningful relationships and activities.
_____	_____	I am committed to at least one project that will improve the quality of life for someone else.
		FOR MARRIEDS ONLY
_____	_____	I give compliments to my spouse several times each day and frequently express genuine gratitude.
_____	_____	I share feelings of anger and frustration directly with my spouse and attempt to resolve conflicts.
_____	_____	I frequently reaffirm my commitment to my spouse and periodically clarify and renegotiate the details of our covenant with him/her.
_____	_____	I set aside time regularly, as well as on special occasions for my spouse and me to invest in our caring relationship.
_____	_____	I forgive my spouse readily and without resentment.
_____	_____	I am willing to postpone the fulfillment of some of my needs and dreams for myself in order to allow my spouse to be more fulfilled.

Count up your "yes" responses for each category and record below:

Family	_____"Yes" responses
Neighbors	_____"Yes" responses
Creation	_____"Yes" responses
Singles or Marrieds	_____"Yes" responses
Total	_____"Yes" responses

PERSONAL REFLECTIONS ON MY WELL-TO-DO PATTERNS

Please answer these questions on the reverse side or blank paper.

- ☐ In what areas are your current outreach investments adequate?
- ☐ In which areas are you neglecting your responsibility?
- ☐ In which areas would you like to increase or decrease your investment in others?
- ☐ Which specific habits would you like to modify?

TRAINER'S NOTES

45 SICKNESS BENEFITS

Participants use a seven-step process to track down the "benefits" they may gain from their sickness or its symptoms. They then identify more responsible alternatives for getting their needs met.

GOALS

1) To identify personal sickness patterns and their origin.

2) To explore the benefits of being sick -- what participants gain from their illness or symptoms.

3) To promote personal responsibility for health.

GROUP SIZE

Works well with a group of 10-12; with a larger number break into 4-6 person discussion groups.

TIME FRAME

10-15 minutes; not more than 20

MATERIALS NEEDED

"Sickness Benefits" worksheets for all participants

PROCESS

1) The trainer introduces the concept of personal responsibility for health and raises the issue of secondary gains -- the rewards received from sickness or its symptoms. She may want to include one or all of the following points:

   - Often we learn in childhood that when we are hurt or ill, we get the attention we crave. Since this care-giving is a powerful reinforcer, we often bring this pattern with us into adulthood, unconsciously striving to get attention through pain or sickness. For many, physical pain or incapacity is preferable to feeling abandoned or unloved!

   - Getting in touch with the "rewards" we are getting out of our pain often helps us to let go of this process. It also allows us to develop more positive ways of getting our needs met as we deal with the stresses and strains of our lives.

- For a child, pain or illness may also be a way to avoid or escape from unpleasant or frightening life situations. Again, we may unconsciously carry this pattern into adulthood and "create" symptoms of illness in order to escape from potential trauma or discomfort.

- Is every cold or broken wrist a plea for attention or an escape mechanism? Probably not! But these may very well be powerful hidden motivators.

2) The trainer distributes "Sickness Benefits" worksheets to all participants, and asks them to begin at the top, listing all the symptoms, illnesses or accidents they have experienced in the past month.

   Note: *The trainer will need to offer several examples to help participants stretch their concepts of "symptoms" and "illnesses" (eg, fatigue, headache, sprained ankle, gas, blisters, stiff neck, hayfever, cancer). Don't forget mental, emotional, spiritual or relationship symptoms like crabbiness, loneliness, depression, anxiety, panic, cynicism, guilt, emptiness, etc.*

3) Participants are instructed to select one of these symptoms for an in-depth exploration.

4) The trainer picks a symptom to use as an example and then goes through the trackdown steps one by one, giving illustrations for each step.

   Note: *This process has the most validity when the trainer uses an example from her own life, but the following example will do in a pinch:*

   Symptom: Headache
   Step 1: <u>It feels like:</u> Being stabbed.
   Step 2: <u>It happens:</u> When I've been under too much pressure.
   Step 3: <u>It prevents:</u> Making positive contact, working hard.
   Step 4: <u>It encourages:</u> Isolation, quiet, withdrawal.
   Step 5: <u>It rewards me with:</u> Sympathy, rest, quiet time alone.
   Step 6: <u>It may indicate a deeper need for:</u> Attention, independence, letting go
   Step 7: <u>A more direct way to meet this need might be:</u> Set limits, say no, articulate my needs.

5) Participants are directed to apply this same process to the symptom they have selected.

6) The trainer summarizes:

- Taking responsibility for our own actions, even our own illnesses, is a giant step towards developing more positive lifestyle habits.

- Recognizing the often-hidden messages behind seemingly common and everyday aches and pains can give us the power to begin changing those symptoms that victimize us.

7) The trainer invites participants to look over their sickness benefits and make a personal resolution concerning their symptoms that helps them take more direct responsibility for them.

8) The trainer asks for reflections, comments, and insights from the group. Participants may read their resolution out loud if they choose.

VARIATIONS

- After Step 7, participants could pair up or form small groups to share their insights and resolutions.

TRAINER'S NOTES

Sandy Queen contributed this process which uses the basic outline of an exercise from John Travis' Wellness Workbook (Berkeley CA: Ten Speed Press, 1981).

SICKNESS BENEFITS

Illnesses, Accidents, Symptoms:

____________________	____________________	____________________
____________________	____________________	____________________
____________________	____________________	____________________
____________________	____________________	____________________
____________________	____________________	____________________
____________________	____________________	____________________
____________________	____________________	____________________
____________________	____________________	____________________
____________________	____________________	____________________

Trackdown Steps:

Choose one symptom/sickness/accident: ____________________

Step 1. It feels like:

Step 2. It happens when:

Step 3. It prevents:

Step 4. It encourages:

Step 5. It rewards me with:

Step 6. It may indicate a deeper need for:

Step 7. A more direct way to meet this need might be:

My resolution:

46 WHEEL OF HEALTH

This extended process helps participants explore the concept of wholeness by involving them in the building of a whole person model and examining the implications of their design. The process includes 3 parts: A) building the wheel model on the blackboard; B) exploring the implications of the wheel; C) Self-examination using the wheel as a personal radar screen.

GOALS

1) To expand participants' awareness of the interconnectedness between all aspects of health.

2) To provide participants with a model for understanding and describing wholeness.

3) To provide participants with a tool they can use to assess their total health.

4) To stimulate the search for creative, non-linear remedies which do not directly tackle the perceived problem.

GROUP SIZE

15-150 persons -- a group smaller than 15 may have difficulty maintaining creative energy to complete the model. A group size of more than 150 makes it difficult for participants to be heard.

TIME FRAME

Approximately 60-90 minutes or more.

MATERIALS NEEDED

A large blackboard that can be seen by all, chalk and copies of the "Wheel of Health" worksheet.

PROCESS

A) BUILDING THE WHEEL MODEL -- A TOTAL GROUP ACTIVITY (20-30 minutes)

1) The trainer introduces the concept of wholeness.

- Neat distinctions which our vocabulary helps us make between body, mind and spirit, simply don't correspond to the reality that we are whole, and that both wellness and illness always involve the total "us" in that process.

- It's difficult to define and grasp this interconnectedness of the whole.

2) The trainer draws a small circle in the center of the blackboard and divides it into five equal parts representing the five dimensions of health -- physical, emotional, spiritual, intellectual and relational, putting a symbol in each.

Physical (Body)
Relational (Two People)
Spiritual (Candle)
Emotional (Heart)
Intellectual (Light Bulb)

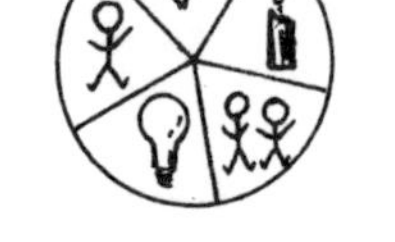

Note: Be sure to tell the group what the symbols stand for. Use your own symbols if you like.

3) The trainer draws a circle around the symbols, extending the lines for each dimension and labels this circle "symptoms."

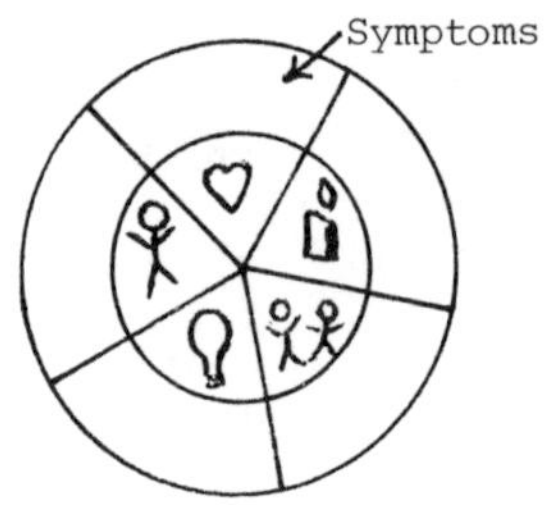

The trainer then selects one portion of the circle and asks the group to suggest symptoms in that area:

- ☐ What are physical symptoms (signs) that something is wrong?
- ☐ What are emotional symptoms? Spiritual symptoms? Intellectual symptoms? Interpersonal symptoms?

The trainer writes down 3-4 suggestions, then moves to the next, until the group has generated symptoms for each area of health.

Note: The trainer should repeat every suggestion of the group while recording it on the blackboard. This reinforces the idea and allows all to hear it!

The trainer should be totally agreeable -- accept whatever symptoms people suggest with no judgment and put the word wherever they tell you. If someone in the group disagrees and argues that the symptom should go elsewhere, ask "Where?" Then put it there also!

4) The trainer then draws another outer ring and labels it "causes".

The trainer as before, asks for 3-4 suggestions from the group -- except now the questions are:
- ☐ What are physical causes for any disease?
- ☐ What are emotional causes? Intellectual causes? Relational causes? Spiritual causes?

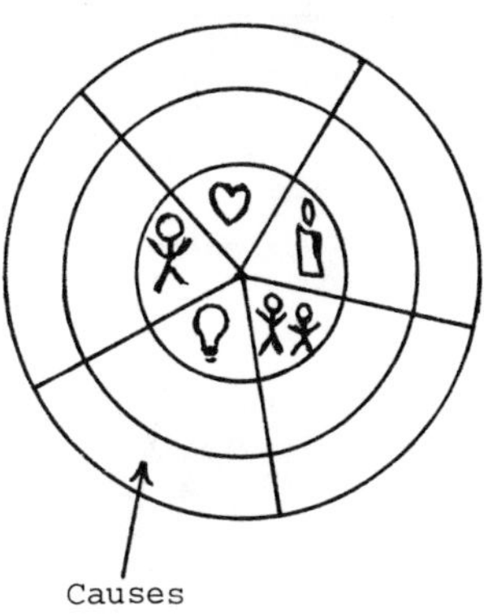

All suggestions are acknowledged and recorded on the blackboard.

Note: Don't look for causes to match the symptoms already in the circle -- just solicit any possible causes.

5) The trainer draws a third ring and labels it "treatments". The questions are:
- ☐ What are physical treatments for any disease?
- ☐ What are emotional treatments? Spiritual? Intellectual? Relational?

Again, all suggestions are acknowledged and recorded on the blackboard.

Note: It is not necessary for the treatments suggested to correspond to the causes or symptoms already listed -- any treatment ideas will do.

6) The trainer draws a fourth ring and labels it "signs of wellness". The questions are:
- ☐ What are physical signs that all is well?
- ☐ What are emotional signs? Spiritual? Intellectual? Relational? etc.

Again, all suggestions are acknowledged and recorded on the blackboard.

B) EXPLORING THE IMPLICATIONS OF THE WHEEL (15-30 minutes)

1) The trainer steps back and looks at the board, while asking the participants, "What ideas or insights occur to you about what we see here?"

   The trainer gathers and acknowledges all points made and continues to ask "what else?", until the group offers no more.

2) The trainer may want to make sure some or all of the following issues surface. Any of these concepts could also be developed in greater depth.

   - Everything is interconnected. Any word could be placed in any segment of health/illness (physical, emotional, etc). Any word could be placed in any ring (symptoms, cause, etc).

     Note: To demonstrate this point further, the trainer can use the following mini-exercise. Choose one person from the audience to write down a symptom, another to select a cause, a third to select a treatment, and a fourth to select a sign of wellness -- all at random. Have each person choose secretly.

     Then ask each person to reveal his selection. The trainer writes these in the corner of the blackboard saying, "Here's a fictional person who experiences ________ (symptom), caused by ________, the treatment utilized was ________ (treatment), and the result was ________ (sign of wellness)".

     The trainer asks whether anyone in the group can describe someone they know who demonstrates that this random combination of factors could be true -- and invites those who respond to tell how this constellation has occurred for them or someone they know.

     Experiment with this mini-exercise two or three times. Since the words describe human experience, no combination will ever be too far fetched.

     Implications? Really, we are one single system -- a whole. We use many words to describe sickness and wellness within different components of our life, but this varied vocabulary is for our own convenience. The words are syntactical fiction. In reality various sicknesses are all connected by a common factor. Sickness is a disruption of wholeness in whatever form it occurs, and healing is a return to wholeness by whatever means.

- Services are disconnected. Our society has dissected individual health into segmented components and developed a variety of separate helping disciplines each of which approaches people primarily from one single viewpoint.

  The results?
  * Separate professional training schools, degrees and licensing regulations.
  * Each discipline learns and develops its own "foreign language" for communicating with peers -- a language that is not understood by those in other disciplines (our modern Tower of Babel?) Labels end up dividing us!
  * Each local community constructs buildings dedicated primarily to healing only one aspect of the person (mental health centers, churches, libraries, hospitals, clinics, YMCA's, health clubs, etc).

- Individuals select symptom patterns. Most people develop a personal pecking order of symptoms -- some symptom areas they want to avoid at all costs, other areas they define as "Okay for me to have symptoms". Unconsciously, people manipulate their description of and attention to symptoms according to their preferences. (For example, one person doesn't mind feeling discouraged and lonely as long as she feels strong physically. Another would never want to lose mental sharpness and concentration, but is more willing to experience physical pain.)

  Note: To illustrate this point further, the trainer may ask the group to mentally rank the symptom areas according to acceptability for them -- "If you must experience symptoms of disease, which area is most okay? Which next most okay? Which is least acceptable to you?" Ask people to compare notes with a neighbor (2 minutes) and then ask the total group to vote by a show of hands for the most acceptable symptom area. Ask about physical symptoms last. About 60% of Americans raise their hands for physical symptoms. What does that mean?

- Individuals develop remedy patterns. Most people also develop a pecking order of personal remedies as well.

Note: To illustrate this point further, the trainer may ask the participants to make a list of their favorite remedies. Then ask how many rely primarily on physical remedies (exercise, diet, drugs), versus other potential options.

- Providers are selected for comfort level. Most people, when they need outside assistance from a professional helper, seek one who by training and license "promises" to define the problem and select the treatments most compatible with their own internal pecking order. In our society, most people are more comfortable with the physical dimension of life. So we define our problem in physical terms and seek physical treatments from a physician. An unspoken silent agreement is formed through this selection process -- "let's deal with this problem physically!"

  What happens when the helper "breaks" the "agreement?" What happens . . .
  * When the physician asks, "How is your marriage?"
  * When the minister asks, "How is your body working?"
  * When the professor asks, "Do you have a purpose beyond yourself?"

  What happens? Usually clients/patients/parishoners -- resist!

- In fact, non-linear treatments are effective. If one imagined spinning the treatment wheel, then stopping it at random -- it is possible that any treatment could be helpful in bringing a return to wholeness in response to any problem.

  This fact illustrates the need for creative, non-linear thinking in the search for remedies, rather than the rational, logical (physical treatments for physical symptoms, spiritual treatments for spiritual problems, etc) problem-solving approach most commonly utilized by every profession.

  The creative wholistic approach opens up a wide range of alternatives not normally considered in the treatment process.

- Wholeness is a process. The wheel is a snapshot of an organism at one moment. In reality we as people have a history, and are moving chronologically across the blackboard through time in an ever-changing pattern.

We are always in process, never static. We are always in one way or another "falling apart" and at the same time in other ways "pulling ourselves together" as we struggle for personal balance and wholeness.

- Wholeness is cosmic. With a few word changes, the wheel, constructed for an individual person could easily stand for a community of family, friends, neighborhood, the city, the state, the nation, the world. Could a wheel of wholeness with symptoms, causes, treatments and signs of wellness be constructed to represent the "community" gathered in the training experience at which this model is being discussed?

C) SELF-EXAMINATION USING THE WHEEL AS A PERSONAL RADAR SCREEN (15-30 minutes)

1) The trainer gives each participant a copy of the wheel worksheet on the following page (or any other variation the trainer has constructed). This worksheet represents a personal radar screen on which participants can note their trouble spots as well as their sources of energy.

2) Participants are asked to circle the words that currently apply to them and to cross out words that do not apply at this time. They also may add any from the board that fit them right now. (5-10 minutes)

3) Participants are then instructed to look objectively at their radar screen and note the "dead spots" and "alive spots" as well as any patterns or surprises they discover.

4) The trainer asks participants to reflect on the following questions.

Note: Allow ample time to answer each question before moving on.

- ☐ Currently, where do you notice symptoms of dis-ease in your life?
  Where do you usually notice them first?
  How do they spread to other life areas?

- □ How does this dis-ease pattern affect your total functioning as a whole person? How does it limit you? How does it protect you?

- □ Which treatment area is your favorite and most frequently utilized? What remedies are most reliable for you?

- □ What additional treatment approaches could you use to correct your current problem?

  Note: Participants will usually choose treatments that relate directly to the symptoms they are experiencing. Encourage them to consider some creative, non-logical treatment selections from other life areas as well.

VARIATIONS

- The trainer may either cut or expand portions of the process to fit the time available, the purpose of the session and the flexibility of the audience. For example, Part A -- "Building the Wheel Model", can easily stand alone as the major focus for a lecture on wholeness. Parts B and C of the process can easily be contracted or expanded to fit the time available.

- The names of the wholeness circles may be changed.
  - Symptoms become "Signs of Stress".
  - Causes become "Stressors".
  - Treatments become "Energizers".
  - Signs of wellness become "Vitality Factors".

- In work with individuals, the radar screen worksheet can be a creative diagnostic tool. It can point up neglected areas that have not been discussed, as well as areas of personal vulnerability or of particular strength.

TRAINER'S NOTES

WHEEL OF HEALTH

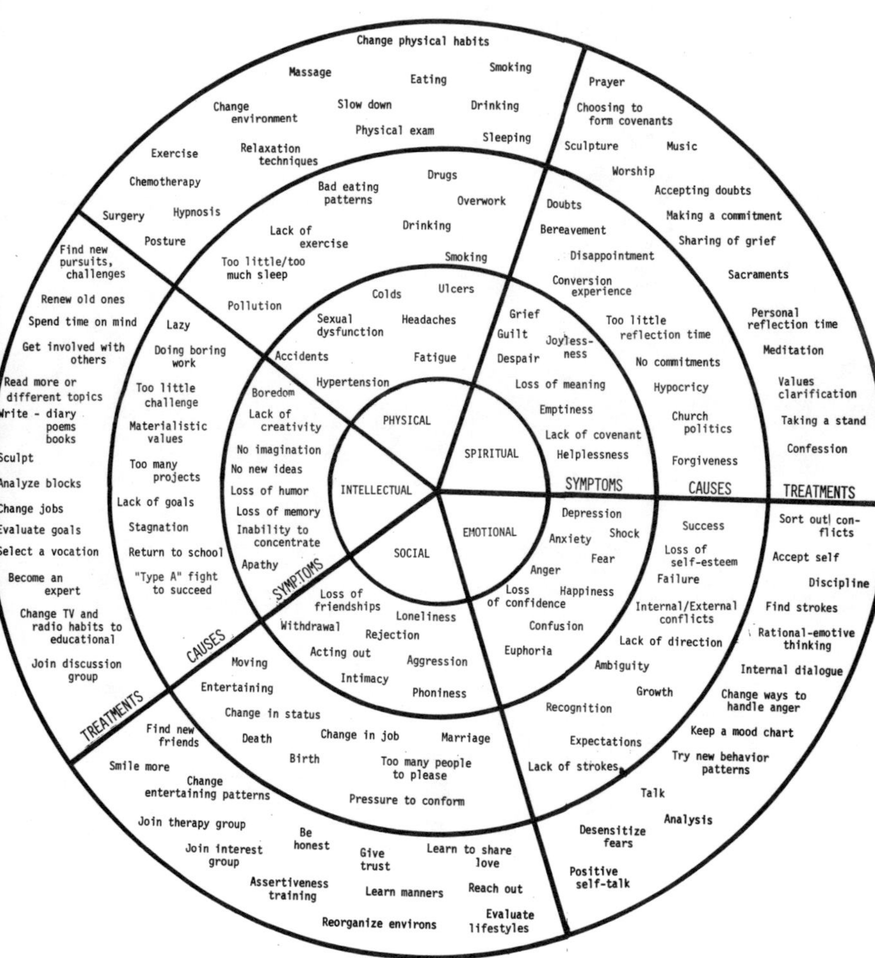

Reprinted from D A Tubesing, Stress Skills Participant Workbook (Duluth MN: Whole Person Associates, 1979).

TRAINER'S NOTES

SELF-CARE STRATEGIES

47 SELF-CARE LEARNING CONTRACT (p 49)

Using a clear and concise goal-setting document designed for a several-session wellness course, participants commit themselves to the course and assume personal responsibility for whatever changes they wish to make.

48 WISH LIST (p 52)

This simple idea can be incorporated into the closure process for each content segment. Participants record all their dreams and hopes about how they could utilize what they have learned to improve their well-being.

49 ANNUAL PHYSICAL (p 54)

Participants draw "real body" and "ideal body" portraits of themselves to highlight their physical assets and liabilities as well as to help them identify self-care goals.

50 LUNCH DUETS (p 57)

Participants pair up for a leisurely meal that accents the process of eating.

51 PERSONAL FITNESS CHECK (p 62)

Participants use a fitness checklist and attitude assessment to pinpoint exercise goals. This process is punctuated by group brainstorming of the obstacles to success and possible strategies for overcoming them.

52 MEDICINE CABINET (p 68)

In this change-of-pace exercise, participants' attitudes toward self-care are explored through an examination of the contents of their medicine cabinets and cosmetic bags.

53 THE POWER OF POSITIVE THINKING (p 72)

This unusual exercise graphically demonstrates the close interplay of the mind/body relationship.

54 LONELINESS LOCATOR (p 74)

This major theme expander challenges participants to distinguish being "alone" and being "lonely," as they explore the theme of dependency in their relationships and plan ways to deal more constructively with their loneliness.

55 COMPASS (p 75)

This do-it-yourself diagram and reflection process helps participants uncover the relative importance of work, relationships, play and the spirit dimensions of life.

56 LIFE AND DEATH QUESTIONS (p 85)

This thought-provoking reflection process helps participants illuminate their spiritual depth and clarify their ultimate purposes which so often are only vague shadows at the edge of awareness.

57 SELF-CARE SOAP (p 89)

In this self-care exercise, participants explore the concept of symptoms as signals and advisors, then borrow a problem-solving process from medical records and apply it to their own symptoms.

47 SELF-CARE LEARNING CONTRACT

Using a clear and concise goal-setting document designed for a several-session wellness course, participants commit themselves to the course and assume personal responsibility for whatever changes they wish to make.

GOALS

1) To secure a personal commitment for change from participants.

2) To activate participants' sense of personal responsibility for their own health.

GROUP SIZE

Unlimited; works well with individuals, too.

TIME FRAME

5-10 minutes

MATERIALS NEEDED

One "Self-Care Learning Contract" for each person.

PROCESS

Note: This exercise is most effective in the first meeting of a multiple-session course focused on promoting lifestyle change. The contract could easily be modified for use in a one-day workshop as well.

1) The trainer distributes the self-care learning contract and highlights the basic principles of taking personal responsibility for health.

2) Participants follow along as the trainer reads and elaborates on the contract.

3) The trainer asks people to think about their reasons for coming to the course, giving examples of some possible motivators (eg, "I'd like to live longer", "I'm overweight", "My blood pressure is too high", "I'd like to feel better", etc).

   Participants are instructed to write down some of the goals they would like to reach during the course (eg, learn about balanced diet, lose 20 pounds, learn when to call the doctor, be depressed less often, etc).

4) The trainer asks people to find a partner who will serve as a witness for the contract signing.

Note: If family members are attending the course together, they may want to serve as witnesses (and reinforcers) for each other.

5) The younger person in each pair begins by reading her goals outloud. The partner gives appropriate encouragement ("Good idea!", "Wow, that's super!", "You can do that!") and both people sign the contract.

6) Partners switch roles and repeat Step 5.

7) The trainer may reconvene the group and ask for examples of personal goals, tying them into the overall goals, the content and the timetable of the course.

VARIATIONS

- In Step 4, participants could choose a partner by finding someone with one or more similar goals.

TRAINER'S NOTES

Submitted by Keith Sehnert

SELF-CARE LEARNING CONTRACT

I have voluntarily enrolled in this class as one step toward taking better care of myself.

I FULLY UNDERSTAND THE FOLLOWING:

1) Change is possible.

2) The more I participate, the more I learn.

3) The more I practice, the faster I learn.

MY RESPONSIBILITIES INCLUDE:

1) To attend classes regularly.

2) To complete the required assignments.

3) To alter my lifestyle in order to achieve the goals listed below.

4) To cooperate in the follow-up program after classes.

I am committed to assuming responsibility for my own health and well-being. My personal plan is to achieve the following:

GOALS ____

____

____

____

______________________ Name ______________________

(Signature)

______________________ Address ______________________

(Date)

______________________ ______________________

(Witness' signature)

______________________ Phone ______________________

(Date)

48 WISH LIST

This simple idea can be incorporated into the closure process for each content segment. Participants record all their dreams and hopes about how they could utilize what they have learned to improve their well-being.

GOALS

1) To provide participants with a written record of their health-related desires.

2) To facilitate the final goal-setting and planning process.

GROUP SIZE

Unlimited

TIME FRAME

5 minutes at the close of each session.

MATERIALS NEEDED

"My Personal Wish List" worksheet for each participant (created by the trainer to fit the content of the session).

PROCESS

Note: This exercise is especially effective as an integral part of a longer workshop or multi-session course. In a single session course, the length and depth of "wish lists" may be less, but the process is identical.

1) At the end of each content segment, the trainer distributes a copy of the "My Personal Wish List" worksheet to each participant. Participants are instructed to spend 5 minutes recording all the hopes, desires and dreams for health that cross their mind in relation to the topic covered. The trainer informs participants that the ideas need not be practical. In fact, they are encouraged to think creatively, being as wild and fanciful as possible in their wishes.

   Note: The trainer will need to provide different worksheets for use at the close of each session. Make the worksheet content specific. The example below is for physical health and could easily be modified for other broad content areas (mental, spiritual, interpersonal health) or specific areas (nutrituion, exercise, relaxation, self-esteem, etc), depending on the course content for that segment.

A WISH LIST FOR MY PHYSICAL HEALTH

Write down here everything you can imagine wanting for your physical health. What would you like to be able to do? to look like? to feel like?

Let your imagination run free. Don't limit yourself in any way. The wishes do not have to be practical. Have fun dreaming.

I wish that . . .

1) ______________________________
2) ______________________________
3) ______________________________
.
.
.
14) ______________________________
15) ______________________________

2) At the end of each segment participants gather data, keeping a separate wish list on each session's topic. In the final planning segment of the course, the trainer invites participants to gather all their separate wish lists and read through them, looking for themes and identifying "wishes" they would like to formulate into specific health-related goals.

3) Participants are then led through the steps of whatever goal setting and planning process the trainer has selected. The left over "wishes" can be saved and used for future plans.

TRAINER'S NOTES

49 ANNUAL PHYSICAL

Participants draw "real body" and "ideal body" portraits of themselves to highlight their physical assets and liabilities as well as to help them identify self-care goals.

GOALS

1) To identify physical assets, liabilities and concerns.

2) To increase body awareness.

3) To isolate areas needing more positive physical self-care.

GROUP SIZE

Unlimited

TIME FRAME

30-45 minutes

MATERIALS NEEDED

Blank paper, writing utensils

PROCESS

1) The trainer distributes blank paper to all participants. The trainer sets the tone by asking people to remember the last time they looked in the mirror -- and to focus on the image in that reflection, asking the questions:

   - What did you see?
   - Did you like what you saw?

   Few people are satisfied with the feedback they get from a mirror.

2) The trainer invites participants to consider themselves as physical specimens, asking them to reflect on questions like:

   - What aspects of your body are you particularly proud of? (beautiful eyelashes? bulging biceps?)
   - What aspects of your physical self are less attractive or at best merely functional? (heavy thighs? short neck?)
   - What physical problems do you carry around with you? (diabetes? a trick knee?)

3) The trainer then directs people to draw a picture of their body. Participants should be encouarged to expand and embellish their drawings, highlighting the weak trouble spots -- the vulnerable areas and limitations they try to hide or protect.

Next, they identify their physical assets and attributes about which they feel particularly proud. They record these on their drawing by using symbols that clearly distinquish these "special glories" from their trouble spots.

Note: No one has to be a Leonardo da Vinci! This is not an art contest. Reassure people that the symbols and insights that come to mind are more important that the drawing itself.

4) The trainer suggests that a mirror is not the only source of feedback about the body. A second and just as important source is the internal stream of signals the body continually sends.

5) The trainer instructs participants to look inside themselves and pay attention to the signals their body sends them -- the stiff neck, the shudder of dread, high blood pressure, the queasy stomach, the energetic eyes, the heartfelt anticipation, the coordination and strength in the legs, etc. Participants then are asked to record their discoveries and sensations on their body picture.

Note: For this step, ask participants to exchange writing untensils with a neighbor so they can distinquish their notes about their internal feedback from the symbols they've already recorded for their external observations.

The trainer may ask questions that focus on the internal body signals like those below, and invite people to embellish their drawings by including pictures or symbols of their responses.

- ☐ Where are the tension spots in your body?
- ☐ What about aches and pains?
- ☐ Are there any areas of concern -- body parts you're worried about?
- ☐ Where is the center of your vitality located?
- ☐ Where do you feel joy? . . . humor? . . . love?
- ☐ What area of your body will be host to your next illness?
- ☐ What part of your body is most well?

6) Once everyone has completed her drawing, the trainer asks participants to turn the paper over and draw a picture of the physical ideal they would like to reach. The trainer may want to ask the following questions one at a time:

- What kind of body are your dreaming about?
- What do you want to be able to do with it? To have it do for you?
- What changes will you have to make in order to reach these goals?
- In what ways does your ideal body picture differ from your "real body" drawing?

7) Participants return to their small groups, or form new groups of 4, and share their pictures and insights with one another.

VARIATIONS

- Participants may make their drawings on large newsprint sheets, using magic markers or crayons. The self-portraits and "ideal" portraits could be hung around the room or taken home to post on the bathroom door as a reminder of self-care concerns.
- If time is short, the internal and external inventories could be combined and participants could pair up to share pictures and insights.
- As a warm up for Step 5, BODY SCANNING, p 113, could be utilized.

TRAINER'S NOTES

50 LUNCH DUETS

Participants pair up for a leisurely meal that accents the process of eating.

GOALS

1) To heighten participants sensory awareness of eating.

2) To explore personal eating patterns.

GROUP SIZE

Unlimited as long as the environment is spacious and comfortable enough for dyads to spread out and feel a sense of privacy.

TIME FRAME

2 hours; could be condensed to one hour with some loss of impact.

MATERIALS NEEDED

Tray of bite-sized food morsels of varying tastes and textures. There should be enough samples of each food so that all participants can get a taste of each variety.

PROCESS

Note: This exercise works most effectively when conducted during a meal time. Participants should bring a sack lunch (breakfast, dinner or snack) to this session.

1) To get the group warmed up to the issue of sensory awareness in eating, the trainer asks a series of questions and uses the data generated as a platform for describing the issues to be considered during the session.

   □ How many people here enjoy eating?

   - Great! Eating is and should be a pleasurable experience.

   - People often overlook one of the primary satisfactions of eating -- the pleasurable sensations associated with tasting, feeling, sucking, slurping, chewing, mushing and swallowing our food. Oral satisfaction doesn't stop with weaning. Just like infants, we derive pleasure from the process of feeding.

- Most of us waste a good share of this sensory pleasure because we don't really taste or feel or play with our food. We're too busy talking, reading, watching TV, arguing, "relating meaningfully", worrying about the next course, counting our calories, etc. We just don't pay attention -- and therefore lose out on a fabulous source of gratification. This exercise will give us an opportunity to pleasure ourselves with the process of eating.

□ How many people have overeaten on occasion -- continued to eat when you felt "full"? How many later regretted that overindulgence?

- We hear a lot about this dynamic -- and do a lot of shaming ourselves when we override our body's signals of fullness and overindulge.

- Paradoxically we do this, not because we enjoy eating so much, but because we don't enjoy it enough! We aren't in the habit of paying close attention to what is satisfying to our bodies! No wonder we don't notice when we've eaten enough to "fill" us! When we start to tune into the pleasurable body signals of eating -- the aromas, tastes, sights, textures, sounds and feel of our food, then we begin to know what is truly satisfying and thus "know" with our bodies as well as our consciences when we've had enough.

□ How many people have ever been hungry?

- Of course we all experience hunger. But since we tend to ignore our body's signals, we often misinterpret their messages.

- When we "feel hungry", we may not be craving food at all! Instead our body may be yearning for a specific physical sensation, (eg, the feeling of something warm sliding down our throat, the satisfaction of grinding our molars together, the stimulation of licking something sticky off our lips, the tension of puckering our mouth around a pickle, the excitement of carbonated bubbles exploding inside our mouth and thousands of other pleasurable sensations that accompany eating.

2) The trainer announces that the remainder of the session will be devoted to rediscovering the sensory pleasures of eating. She asks participants to think about what foods are really pleasureable for them.

After a moment to reflect, she asks for examples of pleasurable foods and for each suggestion probes the specific sensory satisfaction the participant experiences from it, using clarifying questions like the following:

- □ What is particularly satisfying? How it looks? The aroma? The taste (sour, sweet, salty, etc)?
- □ Do you like the sound it makes? The temperature? The texture? The way it feels?
- □ Where do you particularly feel the pleasurable sensation of this food? In you ears? teeth? throat? belly? chest? tongue? lips? gums? All over your body?

3) One at a time, the trainer distributes to the group small portions of four foods with varying tastes and textures (eg, carrot, banana, salted nuts, yogurt, cheese slice, freshly baked bread, raisins, etc). Everyone takes a sample to test for sensory satisfaction.

Participants are instructed to make note of the sensations they experience while slowly eating each different item.

Note: For each food, the trainer may want to suggest that participants inspect it visually, smell it, roll it on the lips, push it around with the tongue, chew with back and front teeth, tuck it under the tongue, mash it against the roof of the mouth, just let it sit, play with it and eventually swallow it. This should be a very slow process.

After each food sample, the trainer solicits comments and insights from the group, asking questions like:

- □ What was most enjoyable about this food?
- □ Where were you most aware of sensation?
- □ What did you notice about the taste and texture?

After all foods are sampled, the trainer asks participants to vote for the most sensory-satisfying food.

4) The trainer announces the the "hors d'oeuvre course" is now completed and it is time to move on to the main meal.

Participants are directed to find someone else in the group with whom they would like to eat lunch (breakfast/dinner/snack). After everyone has found a partner, the trainer describes the process.

Partners are to take their sack lunches, find some private space in the room and eat lunch together, observing a few simple rules:

* Only one person eats at a time. The younger person eats first.
* Each person will have a period of 45 minutes to eat his lunch.
* No one feeds himself. The other person is responsible for feeding her partner whatever he asks for from his lunch.
* The "eater" is to focus full attention on the sensory pleasure of eating, savoring and exploring with all senses each bit of food and drink. He should take small bites, play with the food and experiment with different ways of pleasuring himself while eating.
* Before asking for a food, the "eater" should pay attention to the sensations he wants to experience, and let that awareness guide his choice.
* This is not the clean plate club! Eaters are to eat only as much as pleasures them.
* During this process, partners may talk about what they are experiencing and share any images or memories that are evolked by the process, but idle conversation will distract the eater from his primary focus of sensory awareness and pleasuring.

After 45 minutes, the partners switch roles. This time the older person is fed on request by the younger person, taking a full 45 minutes to enjoy lunch.

Note: The trainer may need to repeat and reinforce the guidelines to incredulous participants (eg, "Yes, 45 minutes -- take your time with each mouthful!" "No, you cannot feed yourself -- your partner will feed you." "Notice what goes on inside you. Talk with your partner about what you are experiencing, but don't distract yourself from paying attention to your sensations!", etc).

5) The trainer reconvenes the large group and facilitates a group discussion about sensory awareness and the process of eating. If the following issues do not come up spontaneously, the trainer may want to ask about:

   * The variety of textures, tastes, etc people brought in their lunches.
   * What people noticed about their styles of eating.
   * How slowing down the pace of eating affected the meal and the pleasure.
   * What were the most sensory-satisfying ways of eating/playing with food?

* How did the imagined or expected pleasure of a food compare with its actual pleasuring power?

6) The trainer asks for closing comments on the implications and applications of what participants experienced during the session.

TRAINER'S NOTES

51 PERSONAL FITNESS CHECK

Participants use a fitness checklist and attitude assessment to pinpoint exercise goals. This process is punctuated by group brainstorming of the obstacles to success and possible strategies for overcoming them.

GOALS

1) To evaluate personal fitness patterns and identify desirable changes.

2) To explore new activity options and attitudes toward them.

3) To uncover and neutralize resistance to aerobic exercise.

GROUP SIZE

12-30 people

TIME FRAME

60 minutes

MATERIALS NEEDED

Copies of the "Personal Fitness Checklist" and "Activity Attitude Analysis" for all; chalkboard or flipchart.

PROCESS

1) The trainer begins by asking a series of questions on which participants "vote" by raising their hands.

   - ☐ How many of you believe that regular exercise should be a number one priority?
   - ☐ How many people in this group exercise vigorously three times per week or more?
   - ☐ How many of you are not exercising currently, but "know" that you should?
   - ☐ How many of you have talked with your physician about exercise?

2) The trainer distributes the "Personal Fitness Checklist" to all participants and asks them to read the statements at the top and check those that apply to them. Participants then answer the questions at the bottom of the worksheet.

3) The trainer again asks for a show of hands on the following question:

- How many of you are genuinely happy with your present activity habits and physical fitness level?

Note: The trainer should reinforce those determined souls who are content by cheering "Bravo!". Invite them during this exercise to act as consultants to their neighbors who would like to begin exercising more regularly.

4) The trainer reminds the group that the evidence is clear -- regular exercise is a positive counter against most coronary heart disease risk factors. If the experts promise that we will feel better, look better, perform better and possibly live longer, why in the world don't we get moving?

The trainer asks the group to share some of the reasons why people (including themselves!) don't exercise more, even when they know it should be a priority. As participants suggest excuses, the trainer restates the roadblocks and writes them on the board.

When the list has grown to 40 or more barriers, the trainer invites the groups to comment on the themes that they see in the list.

5) The trainer then poses a challenge to the group:

- What do these complaints and excuses teach us about designing an aerobic program that will work?

- What do we need to build into an exercise plan so that we are motivated to follow through on our good intentions?

As the group generates ideas, the trainer connects each one to a specific obstacle or complaint and rephrases it as a general principle, using a format similar to the examples given below.

OBJECTION	COUNTERACTION PRINCIPLE
"It's inconvenient"	Make it as convenient as possible (try an exercise "date" for lunch).
"I don't have time"	Schedule it in as an appointment.
"It's boring"	Make the routine fun -- and keep changing it!

OBJECTION	COUNTERACTION PRINCIPLE
"It's hard to keep up"	Build in a reward system, it takes a long time for the intrinsic rewards of exercise to be satisfying.
"I'm too out of shape"	Start slowly, never exceed a pace that allows you to carry on a conversation.
"I've tried it before and it doesn't work"	Stick with it! It takes 4-6 weeks before aerobic capacity is improved.
"I hate jogging"	Try a different activity (aerobic dance? roller skating?)
"It's painful"	Hold to the "conversation pace rule". Find a less stressful activity (swimming? rowing? climbing the walls? running around in circles?)

Note: The trainer may want to elaborate on the principles and give examples of how they might be applied. This is a good time to call in the "consultants" who can share the tricks they've used to help them to continue their exercise program over time.

6) The trainer asks participants to think about their own activity patterns, or rather <u>in</u>activity patterns. What are their own "reasons" for not exercising more? Each participant writes down 4 or 5 of her personal impediments to fitness.

   The trainer directs participants to consider these impediments one by one and for each to write down a principle they could use to counteract that objection or excuse.

7) The trainer asks how many people put "boring" or "I hate exercise" as one of their objections. (Usually, this will be a majority.) He notes that most people who don't exercise regularly think only of a very narrow range of possible activities.

   The trainer distributes an "Activity Attitude Analysis" form to everyone and invites them to consider their current activity habits and attitudes by checking all the appropriate boxes for each type of exercise.

8) The trainer concludes this exercise by asking participants to write their personal responses to the following questions:

- ☐ What do you notice about your current activity pattern?
- ☐ What exercise would you like to add into your daily or weekly routine?
- ☐ How might you start?
- ☐ What are you willing to commit yourself to?

TRAINER'S NOTES

PERSONAL FITNESS CHECKLIST

The statements below describe how you might be feeling about your body and your activity level. Check the statements that seem true for you. Of course, there are no right or wrong answers.

_____ 1) It is not unusual for me to feel tired during a normal work day.

_____ 2) I have a hard time sleeping at night.

_____ 3) It is not unusual for me to have a backache.

_____ 4) I tire much more easily now than when I was younger.

_____ 5) I weigh more now that when I was in my prime.

_____ 6) I am as active as most people my age.

_____ 7) I get plenty of exercise on the weekends.

_____ 8) I keep in shape by playing different sports.

_____ 9) I don't exercise regularly, but I feel good.

_____ 10) I walk very rarely.

_____ 11) I take the elevator (escalator) rather than the stairs.

_____ 12) I am too busy to exercise on a regular basis.

After finishing this checklist, how do you feel about your activity pattern?

Are there any changes you need/would like to make?

ACTIVITY ATTITUDE ANALYSIS

ACTIVITY	I LIKE IT OR DO IT	IT'S OK	I HATE IT	I'VE NEVER TRIED IT	IT SOUNDS INTERESTING
AEROBIC DANCE					
AQUATIC EXERCISE					
BICYCLING					
BRISK WALKING					
CALISTHENICS					
CANOEING					
CROSS-COUNTRY SKIING					
DANCING					
DOWNHILL SKIING					
HANDBALL					
HIKING					
ICE SKATING					
JOGGING					
JUMP ROPE					
RACQUETBALL					
ROLLER SKATING					
ROWING					
SEX					
SQUASH					
SWIMMING					
TENNIS					
WEIGHT LIFTING					

52 MEDICINE CABINET

In this change-of-pace exercise, participants' attitudes toward self-care are explored through an examination of the contents of their medicine cabinets and cosmetic bags.

GOALS

1) To identify underlying attitudes toward health care and illness care.

2) To highlight the role of Madison Avenue in personal self-care habits.

GROUP SIZE

15-40 people; can be adapted for smaller or larger groups.

TIME FRAME

45-60 minutes

MATERIALS NEEDED

Ribbon and construction paper for creating awards.

PROCESS

Note: Because this exercise requires that participants gather the contents of their medicine cabinets and bring these to the session, the trainer must be able to contact participants before hand.

1) Prior to the session in which this exercise is to be used, the trainer gives participants the following assignment. They are to dump the entire contents of their medicine cabinet (and cosmetic kit) into an unmarked paper grocery bag and bring it with them to the next meeting. Participants are not to select "acceptable items only. They are to put everything in the bag. (Yes, old medications, dusty cough syrup bottles, broken Q-tips, K-Y jelly -- whatever is there!) The more true-to-life variety, the better the exercise.

   Participants are assured that they will not be spotted out individually. They may use masking tape to cover their name on any prescription medication before they bring it to the session.

2) As participants arrive for the session, they place

their unmarked paper bags on a series of long tables set up for this purpose.

3) The trainer introduces this exercise with the following thoughts:

- For personal hygiene and self-care of minor symptoms, everyone keeps a small storehouse of personal remedies.

- There are many hundreds of over-the-counter medicines and cosmetics available. Selling them to us is a multi-billion dollar business.

- We make decisions to purchase beauty aids and personal medications based on our beliefs about health. What we buy can teach us a great deal concerning our beliefs about what makes us sick, and our assumptions on how we return ourselves to wellness.

- In this exercise, without embarrassing anyone, we will explore the self-care attitudes of this group by examining the remedies that we purchase over-the-counter.

4) Participants are each instructed to select at random one paper bag from those on the tables. They are then to open the bag and piece-by-piece place the contents of the bag on the table, arranging them as attractively as possible. Since they are "messing with other people's treasures" they are reminded to be very careful and respectful while completing this task.

Note: The trainer must be sure that adequate table space is provided for arranging the items neatly and keeping the contents of each bag clearly separated from the others. Also, the trainer should see to it that ample space is left around the tables for participants to mingle.

5) The trainer divides participants into 4-6 person groups. Each small group is assigned the task of selecting one "medicine cabinet" from among those on the tables for a special award -- each group is the committe of judges for a different award. (See "Special Cabinet Awards" below for ideas.) The trainer makes these award category assignments randomly.

6) The trainer instructs the small group committees to spend the next 15 minutes completing the following tasks:

- Meet together and determine the criteria on which

they will make their award.

- Examine together the contents of each medicine cabinet that is displayed and determine the winner of their category.

  Note: Committees may give a "booby prize award" for the worst cabinet, as well as their "first place winner" prize.

- Construct an award from the ribbon and/or construction paper provided by the trainer, and attach this award ("county fair" style) to the designated display.

7) The trainer reconvenes the group and one-by-one calls on each committee to announce their award. The committee spokesperson describes their category, outlines their predetermined criteria, and then walks to the award-winning medicine cabinet and points out the reasons why it was determined to be the winner.

8) Following the awards presentation, the trainer facilitates a group discussion of reactions to this exercise and insights stimulated by it. Issues that may be raised include:

   - Personal needs and private self-care rememdies are quite varied.
   - The products purchased reflect underlying attitudes and beliefs. What are the beliefs represented on the tables?
   - Many beliefs about what is essential for regaining health and maintaining vitality are sold to consumers via advertising campaigns. The sale of goods follows this altering of beliefs.

9) At the close of the session, participants return their own articles to one of the paper bags and take them home.

TRAINER'S NOTES

SPECIAL CABINET AWARDS

- The FLORENCE NIGHTINGALE AWARD - (best first aid material).
- The R-E-L-I-E-F AWARD - (best collection of digestive aids).
- The REVLON AWARD - (the most elegant "beauty" aids).
- The PLACEBO AWARD - (the most worthless stuff).
- The PAST DUE AWARD - (the most outdated medicines).
- The IATROGENIC AWARD - (the medicines most likely to make you sick).
- The HEAVY WEIGHT AWARD - (the most diet material).
- The BIC AWARD - (for close shavers).
- The SPACE-CASE AWARD - (the most unusual items).
- The UNCOMMON SCENTS AWARD - (the best smelling perfumes/ colognes).
- The STUFFED UP AWARD - (the best cold remedies).
- The ELIMINATOR AWARD - (items to keep you regular).
- The TROJAN HORSE AWARD - (for planned parenthood paraphernalia).
- The BLUE RIBBON AWARD - (the healthiest overall balance).

(Dream up your own!)

53 THE POWER OF POSITIVE THINKING

This change-of-pace exercise graphically demonstrates the close interplay of the mind/body relationship.

GOALS

1) To help participants explore the mind/body connection.

2) To demonstrate for participants that negative thoughts weaken the body, while positive thoughts give it strength.

3) To provide an energizing break in the lecture/discussion routine.

GROUP SIZE

Unlimited, the more the merrier.

TIME FRAME

5 minutes

PROCESS

1) The trainer demonstrates this exercise with the help of a volunteer. The volunteer stands in front of the trainer with eyes closed, and both arms outstretched, one hand resting lightly on top of the other. First, the volunteer is instructed to recall an instance when she felt very happy, confident and proud. As soon as she has this experience clearly in mind and is feeling its joy, she is instructed to nod her head. The trainer then presses down lightly on the outstretched hands, noting the strength of resistance.

   Next, the volunteer is instructed to recall an instance when she felt depressed and embarrassed -- and wished she could crawl into a hole to hide. As before, once she is concentrating fully on this experience she is to nod her head. The trainer again pushes down lightly on her outstretched hands, noting the weakened resistance.

   Note: Don't send the volunteer back to her seat filled with these negative feelings. Ask for a round of applause (or cheers) for her "courage". After the applause, you might even check the strength of her outstretched arms once again. The strength will have returned. (If it hasn't, you are in trouble!!)

2) The trainer instructs participants to stand, find a partner and complete the exercise as demonstrated. The partner testing the strength of the outstretched arms is instructed to note the variation in resistance strength exhibited in conjunction with the two different mental images. Participants switch roles so each has a chance.

3) After all have completed the exercise, the trainer asks participants for their observations on what they experienced.

   Note: Most people will demonstrate greater arm strength when imaging the positive experience and a weakening of the arms when imaging the negative experience. This observation confirms the point that positive thoughts and feelings have a strengthening effect on the body, while negative thoughts and feelings dissipate energies, leaving the person weaker.

   Invariably, in every group there will be some who contend that the negative image made them stronger (more rigid and uptight?), while the positive image created an arm weakness (more relaxed?). Don't make a big deal of this. You may want to joke, "Well, some of you got the right answer and some of you are wrong." Or you might simply say, "In a room with all this noise, it's hard to concentrate on the image and get a clean experiment." In either case, return quickly to the main point, that the mind does indeed have a demonstrable effect on the body.

4) The trainer may want to extend the discussion by asking questions like:

   - What does this experiment teach us about ways in which our health and illness is connected to our attitudes, feelings, beliefs, and self-talk habits?
   - What are the implications?

VARIATIONS

This exercise could be combined with BOO-DOWN (STRESS I, p 113) and WHISPERS (STRESS II, p 130) for an in-depth look at how mental images affect health.

Submitted by Sandy Queen

54 LONELINESS LOCATOR

This major theme expander challenges participants to distinguish between being "alone" and being "lonely", as they explore the theme of dependency in their relationships, and also plan ways to deal more constructively with their loneliness.

GOALS

1) To differentiate between loneliness and being alone.

2) To explore dependency needs that may contribute to feelings of loneliness.

3) To develop positive strategies for confronting loneliness.

GROUP SIZE

Best with groups of 8-12. For numbers over 20, break into small discussion groups (6-8 persons) for this entire exercise

TIME FRAME

60-90 minutes

MATERIALS NEEDED

"Loneliness Locator" worksheets for all; blackboard or newsprint easel.

PROCESS

1) The trainer asks participants to gather their chairs into a circle and make themselves as comfortable as possible.

   Note: *Steps 3 and 5 may evoke a deep level of sharing. If people in the group don't know one another already, take a few minutes now for brief introductions to warm up!*

2) After outlining the general topic for the session, the trainer suggests that participants get started on the discovery process by remembering a time when they felt lonely. Participants are invited to choose one particular experience of loneliness, close their eyes, and visualize as vividly as possible the details of that situation. The trainer facilitates this reflection by

asking participants to remember details, such as:

- □ Where were you?
- □ From whom were you feeling separated?
- □ What did this experience feel like?
- □ Where did you feel the loneliness in your body?

3) After 2-3 minutes of private imaging, the trainer asks people to open their eyes and return to the present. The trainer then invites people to share the loneliness they located, asking a question like, "Who wishes to share briefly what the experience was like?"

Note: *Depending on the group size and time frame, the trainer may allow many or all participants to respond. Don't force anyone. As people share their stories, highlight the central or recurring themes and note the tone (positive/negative) of the image.*

4) After all who wish to share their images have done so, the trainer asks people to close their eyes and get comfortable once again. This time participants are instructed to remember a time when they felt alone. Again, the trainer suggests that people visualize the experience as vividly as possible, asking questions, such as:

- □ What preceded this situation?
- □ Where were you?
- □ Were you feeling separated from someone?
- □ What did this experience feel like?
- □ Could you feel the aloneness in your body? Where?

5) After 2-3 minutes of imaging, the trainer asks people to return to the here and now, then invites them to share their images and perceptions of being alone. The trainer again highlights the themes and tones of the images participants disclose.

6) As the discussion winds down, the group is asked to compare the two types of situations -- being alone and being lonely. The trainer may ask clarifying questions such as:

- □ In what ways are these experiences similar? In what ways different?
- □ What kinds of feelings are associated with loneliness? With being alone?
- □ Was there a difference between the two in the feeling tone? In what ways?

The trainer lists the characteristics in two columns on the blackboard or newsprint.

Note: *In contrast to the experience of "loneliness" which is often accompanied by the feelings of pain or depression, groups usually characterize being "alone" as a positive experience -- time to be by oneself, to reflect, get centered, find peace. The trainer may need to encourage and highlight this viewpoint.*

7) As the discussion progresses, the trainer turns the focus toward the theme of loneliness and dependence, drawing illustrations from the group to highlight some or all of the following points:

- We usually experience loneliness as a result of being cut off or separated from loved ones.

- It seems to be proportional. The more emotionally dependent we are on another person or persons, the more frequent and intense our loneliness is likely to be.

- Yet dependency is a natural part of human relationships.

8) The trainer distributes "Loneliness Locator" worksheets to everyone and guides them through a reflection on their relationships with the important people in their lives.

In Column 1, participants list several people upon whom they are in one way or another dependent (children, parents, spouse, boss, friend, etc).

The trainer asks participants to rate and record (Column 2) the intensity of their dependence on each person using the following scale:

+ I am influenced by and seek this person's (love/acceptance/approval/support), but I could live without it.

++ I feel really empty when I don't feel this person's (love/acceptance/approval/support).

+++ I feel devastated without this person's (love/acceptance/approval/support), and it almost seems like I couldn't survive without it.

Note: *This rating scale could be listed on the blackboard or newsprint for easy reference.*

In Column 3, participants identify for each person listed several needs that this person meets for them (eg, agrees with me, takes care of me, laughs at my jokes, earns money for me, washes my clothes).

The trainer explains that in important relationships what we want and what we get are often quite different (eg, we want intimacy and get clean clothes; we want sympathy and get advice; we want to be nurtured and get sex without emotional closeness; we want respect and get criticism). Participants reflect on each relationship listed and try to identify what they really want to receive from that person. Responses are recorded in Column 4.

The trainer suggests that whenever our wants and needs in a relationship are not met, we feel frustrated. Again participants consider each relationship, asking and answering the question, "How do I respond when these needs aren't met by the other person?" Responses are recorded in Column 5.

Next, participants are directed to consider how they communicate their needs and wants in each relationship (directly? indirectly? nag? criticize? complain? ask? mental telepathy? hints?). These responses are recorded in Column 6.

The trainer points out that most people do not ask directly for what they want or state their needs clearly. The trainer asks participants to suggest reasons why someone might not communicate their wants and needs (eg, fear of rejection; not wanting to appear vulnerable; lack of self-worth; previous disappointments, etc). Participants are instructed to think of each person on their dependency list and note some of the things that block their own expression of wants and needs in that relationship. Responses are recorded in Column 7.

To summarize, the trainer asks people to study their answers and reflect on their overall patterns of relationship and dependency. After they have done this, they are then to answer the two questions at the bottom of the worksheet:

- □ "How do my dependency patterns relate to my loneliness?"
- □ "What are some of the typical ways I deal with my dependency needs?"

9) The trainer invites participants to share with each other in a group discussion their insights on relationships, dependency needs and loneliness.

10) After 10-15 minutes of general sharing, the trainer asks for one participant who is willing to try an experiment, introducing the process with comments like these:

- People who are stuck in unhealthy relationship patterns usually stay stuck because they can't imagine or are afraid to try any new alternatives.

- Often someone outside the situation can easily see different approaches that might be more effective.

- The people in this group have a lot to offer as consultants to one another.

11) The trainer asks the "volunteer" to focus on one of the "loneliness experiences" he uncovered during this exercise and describe it to the group as fully as possible (including a summary of dependency needs, intensity, communication blocks, etc).

    The trainer asks for another "volunteer" to exchange places with the first volunteer and, while sitting in his chair, to describe the strategies she might use to handle the experience of loneliness he described. A second and third volunteer "consultant" could take the hot seat and describe other possible strategies for dealing with that loneliness.

    Note: This step can be repeated several times, each time focusing on a different person's loneliness experience and giving everyone a chance to swap roles and act as "visiting expert" for someone else.

12) The trainer invites people to return to their worksheet and reconsider each relationship they had listed. In light of all the suggestions generated by the group, participants are to list several strategies they could use to minimize their loneliness. Responses are recorded in Column 8.

13) The trainer once again asks the group to find a comfortable position, to close their eyes and to image an experience of loneliness. When everyone has a vivid image in mind, the trainer instructs them to choose one of their new strategies and imagine using it in the situation, visualizing it working effectively to counteract their loneliness.

14) After 2-3 minutes, the trainer directs participants to bring their awareness back to the present and invites closing comments, questions, insights, etc, using these as a springboard for summarizing the content of the session and bringing closure to the experience.

VARIATIONS

- If the group is larger than 20 and Steps 1-10 have been completed without dividing into smaller groups, the trainer should be sure to divide participants into smaller groups of 6-8 persons for Step 11 -- the brainstorming of strategies for dealing with loneliness.

  First, demonstrate how the chair-switching consultation process is to work. Second, ask groups to select a reporter to record all the ideas generated. Then, allow participants in the smaller groups to be consultants to each other. Before moving on to Step 12, the total group can be reconvened and the ideas from each group shared with the whole.

TRAINER'S NOTES

Submitted by Merrill Kempfert

LONELINESS

1 Persons Upon Whom I Am Most Dependent	2 Rating +++ ++ +	3 What Needs Does This Person Meet For Me?	4 What Do I Really Want From This Person?

How do my dependency patterns relate to my loneliness?

LOCATOR

5 How Do I Respond When My Needs Aren't Met By This Person?	6 How Do I Communicate My Wants/Needs?	7 What Blocks My Expression of Wants/Needs?	8

What are some of the common ways I cope with my dependency needs?

55 COMPASS

This do-it-yourself diagram and reflection process helps participants uncover the relative importance of work, relationships, play and the spirit dimension of life. It provides an excellent lead-in for a discussion of personal life absorptions and priorities.

GOALS

1) To explore four meaning dimensions of life: spiritual, creative, loving and work.

2) To promote discussion regarding the variety of personal priorities exhibited by group members.

GROUP SIZE

Unlimited; this exercise can also be used in work with individuals.

TIME FRAME

30-60 minutes, depending on the discussion time allowed.

MATERIALS NEEDED

Blank paper

PROCESS

1) The trainer instructs participants to place a dot in the middle of a blank sheet of paper. The trainer then gives the following instructions (5-10 minutes):

Note: The trainer may want to use a blackboard, newsprint or overhead projector to illustrate instructions step-by-step as the diagram unfolds. The diagrams below are just samples. Use your own examples.

Please consider the importance of <u>spiritual</u> in your life as well as the <u>amount of energy you put into the spiritual dimension of living</u>.

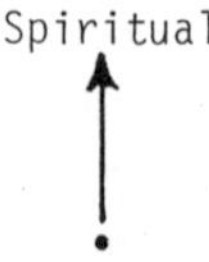

Imagine that the distance between the dot and the top of your page leaves room for a 1-5 scale. Then draw a line from your dot to the top of the page, determining the length of the line according to the level of priority you place on the spiritual dimension of your life.

Consider what activities come to mind as you think of the spiritual dimension and at the top of your page write notes of those images that occur to you.

Please consider the importance of play and creativity in your life, as well as the amount of energy you put into the dimensions of playfulness and creativity.

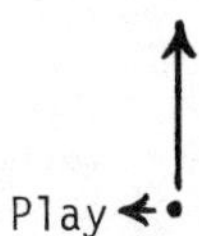

As before, imagine that the distance between the dot and the left side of your page leaves room for a 1-5 scale. Then draw a line from your dot to the left of the page setting the length of the line according to the level of priority you place on the dimension of playfulness and creativity in your life.

At the left hand side of your paper, make a few notes to record the images that occur to you regarding your use of creativity and playfulness.

Please consider the importance of love and loving relationships in your life, as well as your time and energy absorption in fostering and maintaining these relationships.

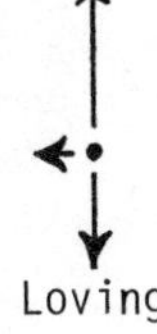

As before, draw a proportional line to the bottom of the page that represents the priority you place on love and loving relationships.

Also, jot a few notes on the bottom of your page to remind you of your loved ones and loving commitments.

Please consider the importance you place on the role of work in your life as well as the amount of time and energy you focus on being responsible, doing a good job and getting ahead in your profession.

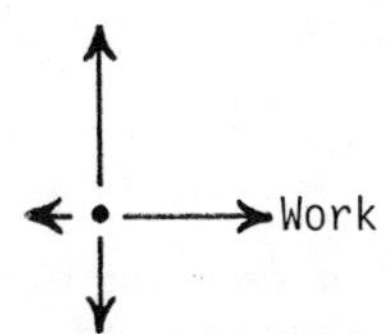

Draw a proportional line to the right of the paper that represents, by its length, the priority level that work and responsibility hold in your life.

Jot a few notes on the right side of the page that indicate your style of approaching the tasks set before you, your focus on work and your feelings of responsibility.

2) The trainer points out that a perfectly shaped diagram is not necessary. Rather this exercise offers an opportunity to view the comparative values assigned to each quality of life.

The trainer asks participants to examine their diagram and their notes carefully, then to write an "essay" that captures the essence of the meaning and purpose in their life as depicted by the diagram they drew. Resistant participants should be encouraged to simply start writing about their observations and feelings and see where the strands of thought take them. (5-15 minutes)

3) The trainer divides participants into groups of four persons each, or utilizes previously formed discussion groups, and invites each person to spend 4-5 minutes describing her diagram as well as sharing observations and insights from her essay. (15-20 minutes)

4) The trainer reconvenes the entire group and may invite the sharing of insights and observations about the exercise and the learnings derived from it.

Note: The trainer may suggest that participants add their insights from this exercise to their personal list of issues to be considered in a later planning process.

TRAINER'S NOTES

This exercise was described to us by Richard Miles, who first read about the idea in Edwin J Kepler's paper on chronic fatigue in the "Proceedings of the Staff Meetings of the Mayo Clinic," Vol 17, No 22, June 3, 1942.

56 LIFE AND DEATH QUESTIONS

This thought-provoking reflection process helps participants illuminate their spiritual depth and clarify their ultimate purposes which so often are only vague shadows at the edge of awareness.

GOALS

1) To help participants clarify their goals, values and beliefs.

2) To incorporate the reality of death into an understanding of whole person well-being.

3) To demonstrate that spiritual health is an essential element of wellness.

GROUP SIZE

Unlimited, this exercise may also be assigned to individuals as between-session "homework".

TIME FRAME

60 minutes (20-30 minutes if the group sharing is omitted).

MATERIALS NEEDED

Blank paper, blackboard or overhead projector.

PROCESS

1) The trainer introduces this centering exercise by outlining some or all of the following spiritual wellness concepts:

   - The mortality rate in this room is 100%. All life is terminal. We cannot get out alive.

   - As part of our movement toward health-fullness we must all come to grips with the meaning of death. Death is not necessarily a defeat. It is the backdrop against which we see life clearly and discover its ultimate meaning for us.

   - Health is related to our choices about integrating death into our view of life rather than playing hide and seek with it. The race against death turns life into a long series of futile attempts to avoid it. This race against death provides no security, no purpose, no values; and makes it impossible for us to get on with the task of choosing how to live. Affirming values and beliefs that encompass death, frees us to live life with clarity and gusto!

- It is tempting to measure life by the wrong standards. Rather than judging the value of life by its length, perhaps we should look instead to the worth of the principles and purposes for which we live. Health-fullness cannot be determined on the basis of whether we live to be 40 or 70 or whether we burn ourselves out early or late.

- Our answers to the question, "Am I spending myself where it counts?" may be the best assessment of our wellness.

- When you can visualize your death occurring at any moment, and can still imagine yourself saying, "I have no regrets. I would live my life the same way all over again", then you have demonstrated the ultimate evidence of well-being.

- You don't have to wait for tragedy or someone else's death to illuminate your life and to indicate for you your personal path toward making health-full choices. This exercise will help you seek your own answers to in-depth spiritual questions:
  * Who am I?
  * What do I stand for?
  * When all the surface layers are peeled away, what is at the core of my life? of me?

2) The trainer instructs participants to select an age at which they feel it will be appropriate for them to die, and to write that number in the center of their paper. (The trainer may facetiously suggest that for obvious reasons, the number they choose should be at least as large as their current age!)

3) Participants are then instructed to draw a circle with their death age number on the circumference, and to draw a radius line from the center of the circle to the number. The trainer will demonstrate this and the following steps on the board or overhead.

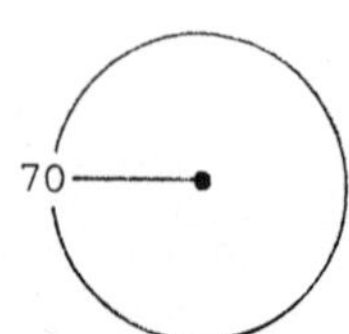

4) The trainer informs participants that the area inside the circle represents the time of their life. She then instructs people to write down their current age at the appropriate point on the circumference, draw a line to it, and then shade in the percentage of the circle that represents the time that they have already lived.

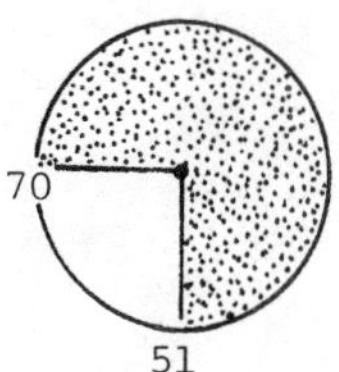

5) The trainer instructs the participants to focus on the time that is left as they answer the next series of questions. The trainer asks the following questions, one at a time, allowing ample opportunity for reflection.

- Imagine that you died in your sleep tonight. What is left undone? Please list as many goals and activities as you can, as quickly as you are able.
- What would you like to have done differently?
- What do you wish you could still say to those you love?
- What positive differences had you still hoped to make in your world?

6) The trainer gives participants a few minutes to reflect on their answers, and encourages them to write down any insights, surprises, disappointments, etc that occur to them as they examine what they've written so far.

7) The trainer then asks a second series of questions, one at a time, instructing participants to write down their answers to each.

- What does facing your death help you see about your major values and purposes?
- What does thinking about your imminent death tell you about how you should choose to live your life from now on?
- Have you been spending yourself where it counts? In what ways "yes" and in what ways "no"?
- Are there any changes you need to make now? What specifically?

- ☐ In light of your values and purposes, please outline an appropriate summary of the goals and activities that should fill the time you still have remaining before your expected date of death.

8) The trainer divides participants into small groups of 3-6 persons (depending on the time available, and the trust level extant in the group) and invites them to share their answers with one another, listening to the personal descriptions of issues confronted, joys experienced and pain faced by participants while they were completing this exercise.

9) The trainer reconvenes the entire group and asks for a sharing of insights and observations. Participants may be asked to respond to the question, "What does all of this serious thinking have to do with wellness?"

   The trainer may also want to challenge the group to "do what they need to do - NOW!" And she may even offer a pocket full of quarters to those who need to rush to a telephone and talk to a loved one.

TRAINER'S NOTES

57 SELF-CARE SOAP

In the first part of this self-care exercise, participants explore the concept of symptoms as signals and advisors. During the second segment, they learn a problem-solving process borrowed from medical records and apply it to their own symptoms.

GOALS

1) To increase participants' understanding of the role of symptoms as warning signals and advisors.

2) To build skill in describing health problems accurately.

3) To provide an easy-to-remember problem-solving tool for health concerns.

4) To motivate participants toward personal self-care responsibility.

GROUP SIZE

12-30 people

TIME FRAME

90 minutes

MATERIALS NEEDED

A copy of the "Self-Care SOAP Worklist" for everyone, blank paper, chalkboard or newsprint easel.

PROCESS

1) The trainer begins the session by asking if anyone is currently experiencing symptoms that are bothering them right now (eg, sore back, headache, sore feet, stomach-ache, stuffy nose). Participants give examples.

   The trainer asks those who shared symptoms to tell others in the class a bit about the problem and what might have caused the symptoms (eg, "I hurt my back shoveling snow", "I have a headache from watching the computer monitor all day", "The baby has a cold and I think I'm coming down with it, too").

2) The trainer uses data generated from these examples to illustrate the importance of symptoms:

- Symptoms can be compared to the gauges and lights on a car's dashboard, which allow us to monitor our progress and warn us of potential problems. They tell us if our tank is full or empty, if the engine temperature is right. They tell us how fast and in what direction we are headed. They even remind us to buckle up.

- The physical symptoms we experience are much like these indicators. Our bodies "talk" to us via these symptoms, keeping us posted on how we're doing and alerting us to problems that may need attention before they get out of hand.

- Symptoms can even give us advice about how to take care of ourselves (eg, pain in the ankle advises us not to put weight on it, fatigue advises us to get more sleep, uncomfortable fullness reminds us to stop eating, etc).

3) The trainer invites participants to experience a series of exercises that simulate common health problems and demonstrate the messages our bodies send us as symptoms.

   Note: The trainer should demonstrate while giving the step-by-step instructions in Steps 4, 5 and 6.

4) To simulate common cold symptoms, the trainer instructs the group to follow these steps:
   - □ Hold your nose.
   - □ With mouth open wide, breathe in deeply 10-15 times.

   The trainer then asks the group what symptoms they noticed (dry mouth? cough? tickle? sore throat?) and writes these down on the chalkboard or newsprint.

   The trainer comments on the lists of symptoms and points out how the exercises altered some body functions which then resulted in uncomfortable symptoms (eg, the nose moistens the air we breathe. With our nose closed, we dry out our respiratory tract.)

5) To simulate sore joints, participants are instructed:
   - □ Raise your right arm straight above your head.
   - □ Open and close your fist as quickly as possible 15-20 times.
   - □ Again, clench your fist as tightly as possible and keeping it tight, lower your hand to your lap.
   - □ Look at the color of the skin on your hand.

The trainer again invites people to share the symptoms they noticed (Sore wrist? Stiff shoulder? Pale skin? Aching fingers? etc). All symptoms are recorded on the board.

The trainer notes that by clenching and elevating our fists, we reduced the blood supply which resulted in paleness and discomfort.

6) Participants are directed in a search for symptoms in the neck area.

- □ Place the fingertips of both hands on the back of your neck, on either side of the spine.
- □ Feel the muscles up and down your neck along the spine. You may want to try different pressures.
- □ Move your fingers to behind your ears and feel up and down your neck in that area.
- □ This time start just under your ears and feel up and down with your fingertips.
- □ Now, start with your fingers under your jaw on either side and feel up and down the front of your neck.

The trainer asks people to comment on the symptoms they discovered (Stiff muscles? Sore spots? Tender areas on the bone? Lumps?) and makes a list of them.

The trainer notes that pain and tightness usually indicate muscle tension, which restricts blood flow. Tenderness might be traced to lymph glands which are swollen in their efforts to drain away infection.

7) The trainer asks the group to give additional examples of symptoms they have experienced at different times or heard other people talk about (eg, pain, distress, fatigue, etc). The trainer notes that most of the symptoms are "bad" signals sent from our bodies that suggest something is "wrong".

8) He reminds the group that our bodies also send "good" signals that indicate "all is well" (eg, satisfaction after a meal, exhiliration after exercise, soothing relaxed sensation after a back rub or snuggling with a child, etc). Participants are invited to give additional examples of "good" signals they have experienced.

9) Participants use blank paper to make a list of the "good" and "bad" signals they experienced yesterday (or this week). (3 minutes)

Note: This is an excellent time to take a refreshment, stretch, or "pit stop" break. The trainer can ask the group if they are experiencing any symptoms right now that indicate the need for a break. (EXERCISES FOR THE SEDENTARY, p 118, would fit well here.)

10) After reconvening the group, the trainer distributes the "Self-Care SOAP Worklists" and introduces the SOAP process, covering the concepts below:

- SOAP is an acronym borrowed from the problem-oriented medical records technique which is used to describe, diagnose and treat health problems.

- S stands for subjective -- the individual's description of the problem. What is bothering you? When does it occur? Where does it hurt? Answers to these and similar questions constitute a medical "history".

- O stands for objective measurements of vital signs and other symptoms, often obtained by using measuring devices such as a thermometer, stethescope, sphygmomanometer, otoscope, fingers, etc. Visual observation, color, size, etc is also objective.

- A stands for assessment -- comparing observations with some external standards such as the "normal" range. A physician can rely on years of training and the experience of seeing many other people with similar symptoms to make this assessment. Self-care advocates need to rely on a reputable self-care text book and phone consultation with health care providers.

- P stands for plan -- determining the best treatment for the symptoms and taking that action. For activated patients this also means the ability to determine what signals will indicate that professional help is needed and should be sought.

11) The trainer announces that the rest of this session will be a skill-building workshop on the S step of SOAPing. The focus will be on subjective data and descriptions of common health problems, using symptoms group members or their families have experienced recently. The trainer asks for "volunteers" who would be willing to have their health concern "SOAPed".

Note: *The next part of the exercise is completed in groups of 5-6 persons each. The trainer needs to decide how many groups there will be and assign one health concern "volunteer" to each group. If too many people volunteer, select problems on the basis of diversity and appropriateness for group discussion.*

12) Participants are divided into groups of 5-6 persons including one volunteer whose real life health problem will be SOAPed by the group. (Each group has a different problem.)

Note: The trainer will probably need to review again the Subjective process for describing symptoms. The prompter words, "What", "When", "Where", "How often", etc may be written in large letters on the board for easy reference in the next step.

13) The trainer instructs the "volunteers" to begin by describing their health problem to their small group. The rest of the group members refer to their "worklists" and are encouraged to ask respectful, clarifying questions (eg, "When did the cold begin?" "What bothered you first?" "Who else has been sick?" "How has it affected your appetite?" "What other experience is this like?" "What other symptoms have you noticed?" etc). The volunteers should be allowed to protect their privacy by not responding to questions that feel uncomfortable. One person in each group acts as recorder, jotting down all the information about the problem and its symptoms as the history unfolds.

14) The trainer reconvenes the large group and asks the recorder from each small group to state the health problem they worked on and a brief symmary of the symptoms that accompanied it.

15) The trainer picks up on the themes revealed in these "histories" and uses them to summarize and illustrate concepts covered during the session.

16) Participants are encouraged to use their SOAP Worklists after the session to problem-solve one of their own health concerns.

VARIATIONS

- This exercise could be transformed into a "whole person" model by expanding consideration of symptoms to include mental, emotional, spiritual or lifestyle signals as well as physical.

SELF-CARE SOAP WORKLIST

SUBJECTIVE: How to describe the problem.

The SOAP process begins with describing the symptoms associated with the problem. Gather as much information or history as possible about how the illness, injury or problem affects the person or makes them feel. Ask questions such as "What started the pain?", "Where is the soreness?", "When does the throat hurt most?", "What concerns you most?".

Stated problem ______________________________

Expanded description

What? ______________________________

When? ______________________________

Where? ______________________________

How? ______________________________

OBJECTIVE: How to measure the problem.

The second step in the SOAP system involves measuring or making observations about things related to the problem. Use the appropriate instrument (including your eyes, ears and fingers) for measuring symptoms, such as:

Temperature ______________
Blood pressure ____________
Pulse (per minute) ________
Breathing rate ___________
Location of swelling ______
Length of cut/wound ______
(inches, centimeters)
Time between pains ________

Color of mucous ___________
Color of urine ___________
Color of ear drum ________
Color of throat __________
Amount of discharge ______
(teaspoon? tablespoon?)
Frequency of diarrhea ____
(times per hour)

What else can you observe about the problem:

____

____

____

____

ASSESSMENT: How to compare the problem.

The third step in the SOAP system involves comparing the symptoms and observations already made and recorded with information from some authoritative source such as a self-care manual organized by symptoms. Look up the symptoms in the index and read about each problem that might cause these particular symptoms. For each potential problem answer these questions:

Have you ever had these symptoms before? ☐ Yes ☐ No
If "yes", describe which ones and when ______________________

____

Are the symptoms the same as the book describes for this problem? ☐ Yes ☐ No
If "yes", please list ______________________
If "no", look up another problem with similar symptoms.

Are the indications you checked or measured the same as those described in the book? ☐ Yes ☐ No
If "yes", please list ______________________
If "no", look up another problem.

PLAN: How to decide on and begin treatment (which may include seeking professional help).

The final step in the SOAP process involves deciding if professional help is, or might be, needed and beginning a home treatment plan. Use a reputable self-care guide or another reliable resource to determine:

Are there any "call the professional" signals present? ☐ Yes ☐ No
If "yes", please list ______________________

What supplies will you need? ______________________
Do you have them on hand? ☐ Yes ☐ No
If "no", please list what is needed ______________________

What is the first step in treatment? ______________________

Please describe the whole plan ______________________

____

When will you seek professional help if the problem doesn't improve? Please set time, circumstances ______________________

____

TRAINER'S NOTES

This exercise is one of five sessions in a health activation program created by Keith Sehnert, author of The Family Doctor's Health Tips (Minneapolis: Meadowbrook, 1981) which is used as a text for the course.

ACTION PLANNING / CLOSURE

58 WHAT NEXT? (p 97)

This simple process for ending a workshop day on a quiet note is particularly appropriate as a mid-workshop dismissal when additional sessions are scheduled for the following day.

59 ROUNDUP REVISITED (p 98)

This quick closing exercise reviews the content and explores participants' satisfaction with the learning experience.

60 CLEANING UP MY ACT (p 99)

This activity is geared for participants who want to "clean up their act" by making several lifestyle adjustments at the same time.

61 ONE-A-DAY PLAN (p 106)

This creative process helps participants formulate a 30-day plan for reaching specific wellness goals.

62 VITAL SIGNS (p 109)

In this powerful closing exercise, participants affirm directly the signs of vitality which they have seen and appreciated in each of the other members of their small discussion group.

58 WHAT NEXT?

This simple process for ending the workshop day on a quiet note is particularly appropriate as a mid-workshop dismissal when additional sessions are scheduled for the following day.

GOALS

1) To slow down the pace and allow participants to focus themselves before leaving the workshop.

2) To encourage integration and application of the day's material.

TIME FRAME

10-15 minutes

PROCESS

1) The trainer asks participants to silently identify for themselves what they plan to do as soon as they are dismissed from the session (eg, drive home, go out for dinner, visit friends, play with kids, go back to work).

2) The trainer explains that she will take the last ten minutes of the session to offer participants a chance to focus inward and be quiet for a few moments before being dismissed. She then leads participants through a short relaxation exercise. BODY SCANNING, p 113, TAKE A DEEP BREATH, p 127, or UNWINDING (STRESS I, p 73) would work well.

3) Following the relaxation exercise, the trainer instructs participants, "Now go and do whatever you imagined you would do when I dismissed you (eg, drive home, go out for dinner, visit friends, play with kids, go back to work). But notice whether you do it differently now, after you've relaxed, than you would have done it had I ended this session ten minutes ago."

4) At the beginning of the first session of the next day, the trainer may ask for a report on what participants experienced.

59 ROUNDUP REVISITED

This quick closing exercise reviews the content and explores participants' satisfaction with the learning experience.

GOALS

1) To give participants an opportunity to compare their original expectations with what they actually gained from the training event.

GROUP SIZE

Up to 25. With larger numbers, divide into groups of 8-10.

TIME FRAME

1-2 minutes per participant.

PROCESS

Note: This is most effective when paired with its companion icebreaker, ROUNDUP, p 1.

1) The trainer asks people to recall the expectations they originally brought to the session/meeting/workshop (and stated in the opening ROUNDUP).

2) Participants are directed to compare those hopes with what they in fact have gained from the learning experience.

   Note: The trainer may want to briefly review the topics covered to stimulate recall.

3) Starting with the trainer, participants fill in the blanks and share their sentence:

   * "My expectation for today's session/meeting/workshop was _________ and what I gained was _________.

   Note: Don't ask for or permit explanations. Do allow people to pass.

4) The trainer summarizes participants' learnings and tells the group how they have been a "special" learning experience for him!

This exercise was adapted from Lois Hart's Saying Goodbye: Ending A Group Experience. (Lyons Co: Leadership Dynamics, 1983)

60 CLEANING UP MY ACT

This activity is geared for participants who want to "clean up their act" by making several lifestyle adjustments at the same time. A unique number system helps people translate selected health-enhancing and health-depleting behaviors into a daily and weekly vitality balance sheet. Participants work to improve their "bottom line" numbers over several weeks.

GOALS

1) To enhance personal vitality by increasing the frequency of positive health behaviors while decreasing the frequency of negative ones.

2) To help participants make incremental lifestyle adjustments one step at a time.

GROUP SIZE

Any size group is appropriate. Individuals may utilize this exercise on their own, although group support and reinforcement help immensely.

TIME FRAME

30-45 minutes for the planning exercise; 5-10 minutes homework per day for the next four weeks.

MATERIALS NEEDED

"Cleaning Up My Act" worksheets and two 3" X 5" notecards for each person; blackboard or newsprint easel.

PROCESS

Note: The instructions for this exercise look complicated, but the process itself is actually quite simple, and well worth the time it takes to understand it. Be sure to try it for yourself before using it in a session. One week of charting your own plus and minus tallies will make the exercise come alive and give you the personal examples you'll need to describe the process effectively.

Some participants will find that the "game" of working to improve their score becomes a reward in itself. They may change health habits for a secondary purpose -- simply to score higher. Whatever the motivation, higher scores should lead to higher vitality. For others, numbers and the "scoring system" will have little appeal. Encourage them to give the process a try anyway!

1) The trainer introduces the exercise with some brief comments on health, vitality and the change process, covering some or all of the following points:

   - We don't have to make massive lifestyle changes in order to feel more lively, vital and healthy. It's the little things that count -- the accumulation of hundreds of health-enhancing and health-depleting behaviors that we engage in daily.

   - We can improve our vitality balance by reducing or eliminating negative behaviors and/or by increasing or adding positive ones.

   - Good health is not just a physical issue. Mental, spiritual and interpersonal self-care habits play an equally important role in regaining and maintaining overall vitality.

2) The trainer invites participants to suggest examples of health-depleting behaviors -- negative habits they might want to stop, or at least decrease (eg, smoking, eating high cholesterol foods, worrying, cynicism, etc). The trainer prompts people to consider "depleters" in all dimensions of life (body, mind, spirit, relationships). Suggestions are recorded on the board until the list reaches at least 50 behaviors.

3) Participants are invited to examine the other side of the vitality equation, suggesting examples of health-enhancing behaviors -- positive habits they might like to continue or increase (eg, tooth-flossing, meditation, walking, high-fiber diet, creative problem solving, regular sleep patterns, etc). The trainer lists all suggestions on the board until the group has generated 50 or more.

4) The trainer announces that the balance of time will be spent in designing personalized plans for change that will help participants alter whatever lifestyle patterns they want to adjust in order to increase their vitality.

   Note: In the following steps, participants may want to refer to the list of changes generated in Step 2, but they should not be bound by it. Each person should reflect on her current lifestyle and construct her own list. Any behaviors that potentially add to or subtract from vitality can be used.

5) Identifying positive target behaviors. The trainer distributes two 3" X 5" index cards to all participants and directs them to divide one side of each card into columns, numbering them 1-4. One card should be labeled "INCREASE" and the other "DECREASE".

Note: The trainer should demonstrate the process of Steps 5-9 on the board. Construct "notecards" similar to the samples below as you go along, but use your own personal examples.

INCREASE (or DECREASE)	*1*	*2*	*3*	*4*
TOTALS	*(importance factor)*	*(typical week frequency)*	*(product)*	*(one week totals)*

The trainer then asks participants to decide which positive health behaviors they would like to increase (eg, naps, contact with friends, eating more vegetables, getting up early, listening to music, writing letters, prayer, exercise, playing with the kids, deep breathing, etc). These targeted behaviors should be activities that are or could be repeated several times a day or week.

Each participant lists 4-5 positive behaviors she would like to increase on her "INCREASE" notecard. Space should be left at the bottom for "TOTALS".

Note: The trainer may need to remind participants that this is an individualized plan, telling the group, "The behaviors you choose to modify will be entirely your own."

6) Determining the "importance factor". Next, participants assign a point value to each item they have targeted for increase. In Column 1 ("importance factor"), they mark a "+1" for minor behaviors they want to increase, a "+2" or a "+3" for those that are a bit more important and a "+4" or a "+5" for those that are the most effective positive behaviors.

Note: If participants turn to you for clarification and guidance, remind them that the point value should be determined solely by each individual based on how important the change is to her and how effective she believes the change will be in increasing her vitality.

INCREASE	*1*	*2*	*3*	*4*
Exercise (20 minutes)	*+5*	**(1)*	**(+5)*	
Phone a friend	*+2*	*(10)*	*(+20)*	
Meditation	*+3*	*(3)*	*(+9)*	
Laugh	*+1*	*(30)*	*(+30)*	
Deep breathing	*+2*	*(12)*	*(+24)*	
TOTAL			*(+88)*	

*To be determined in Step 9

7) Identifying negative target behaviors. After everyone has listed and valued her positive health changes, the trainer instructs participants to use a similar process for charting the negative behaviors they would like to reduce (eg, drinking beer, working through lunch, wasting time, staying up late, using caffeine, worrying, eating junk food, complaining, etc). As before, these changes should be discrete behaviors that are repeated several times a day or week.

Participants fill in their cards, writing down the 4-5 behaviors they are targeting for decrease.

8) Determining the "importance factor". Next, participants decide how to weight each of these changes by designating a point value for each negative behavior. In Column 1 people mark a "-1" for those habits they want to decrease, a "-2" or "-3" for those changes that are more important and a "-4" or "-5" for the most destructive negative behaviors. These values are determined solely by the individual.

9) Estimating a baseline frequency. The trainer invites participants to measure their current patterns by estimating the number of times they engage in each targeted behavior during a typical week. This number is recorded in Column 2 of each card.

Participants multiply the frequency by the "importance" points for each behavior and record the (+ or -) products in Column 3. The "INCREASE" card will show positive totals, the "DECREASE" card negative totals.

The trainer instructs the group to add up their totals in Column 3 for each card to determine the total number of positive and negative points they would typically accumulate in a week.

Note: Make sure that everyone understands this step. If necessary, review the concept of positive and negative numbers, giving several examples.

DECREASE	*1*	*2*	*3*	*4*
Junk Food	*-2*	*21*	*-42*	
Complaining	*-1*	*14*	*-14*	
Smoking	*-1*	*110*	*-110*	
Working through lunch	*-5*	*3*	*-15*	
Staying up after 11	*-3*	*5*	*-15*	
TOTAL			*-196*	

The trainer distributes "Cleaning Up My Act" worksheets and asks everyone to write their plus totals from their "INCREASE" card and their minus totals from their "DECREASE" card in Section A. Participants then compute their "typical week" baseline number as indicated on the worksheet. (For the example here, (+88) + (-196) = -108.)

Note: *The trainer may need to clarify further, saying something like, "This number is your baseline number. Each person's will be different. This number represents your current positive/negative health habit pattern. If you want to make a positive change in this pattern, you will need to aim for a higher number next week. Your success will always be measured in relation to this baseline number."*

10) Goal-setting. The trainer guides the group through the goal-setting process as outlined on the worksheet Section B. He reminds participants that it's the little steps that count up over the long run. The goal they set should be higher than their baseline to represent some "improvement". This improvement can be accomplished by reducing negative behaviors, increasing positive ones, or doing both. The goal should also be realistic.

Note: *Remind participants that their baseline numbers have no real value in themselves. Use a number line to illustrate this point. It's okay to start with a negative number and strive for improvement by targeting for a smaller negative number. Any movement to the right is a movement for higher vitality!*

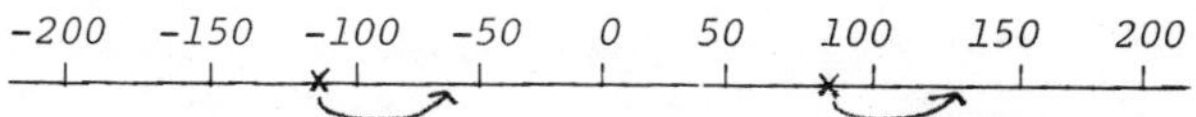

For example, a person currently at "-108" could set her goal for the week at "-60" and still be aiming for significant improvement. Someone with a baseline of "+88" would need to target a number higher than that in order to show improvement.

The trainer may want to encourage participants by saying, "You will measure yourself and your improvement against yourself and your prior patterns. Your neighbor's goals are irrelevant to you. Resist the temptation to compare yourself with others! Simply aim for a goal that represents an improvement for you.

11) Monitoring. Participants are instructed to monitor their behavior for the next week, counting every time they engage in each targeted behavior -- both the positive and negative ones. The trainer elaborates on how the point system can work:

- The trick is to keep a mental or written balance sheet, updating it every day or several times a day. Add up your "+" points. Subtract your "-" points. Then ask:
  * What is my total for the day so far?
  * What is my accumulated total for the week?
  * How am I doing in relation to my goal?
  * What adjustments do I need to make?

- With this system, you don't have to be perfect. You gain points each time you increase a positive behavior or decrease a negative one. You can adjust your behaviors as needed to reach your goal. If you accumulate some extra positives, maybe you can "afford" to lose a few points. If you get yourself into a hole, you can climb out by accelerating the pace of your positives. As long as you are increasing your positive point total over time you will soon begin to experience an increase in your overall vitality.

The trainer notes that each person will have to discover the best way to keep track of her plus and minus points during the day and week (eg, another notecard, diary, calendar, etc).

At the end of the week, totals for each behavior are recorded in Column 4 of both notecards and a final point count for the week is calculated.

12) Evaluating. The trainer encourages participants to evaluate their progress at the end of the week, recording their point totals in Section D of the worksheet.

Note: If the trainer is meeting with participants in a series of weekly sessions, this reporting and reevaluation should be built into the design of each meeting. If not, remind participants to continue the plan on their own for at least four weeks.

CLEANING UP MY ACT

A. FIND A BASELINE:

(+ ________) + (- ________) = ________
Positive total + Negative total = Baseline

B. SET YOUR GOALS

1) Set a goal for the total number of points you hope to reach in a week. Be realistic, but aim for improvement.

   My goal for the week is __________ total points.

2) Imagine ahead. How do you expect to feel health-wise at the end of the week if you reach your goal? __________

   ____

3) Set an appointment with yourself, in exactly seven days to evaluate.

   I will evaluate my progess on ________ (Date) at ________ (Time).

C. MONITOR YOUR PROGRESS ON A DAILY BASIS ALL WEEK LONG

D. EVALUATE YOURSELF AND START AGAIN

At the end of the week, evaluate: My point total for the week is ________.

* How did it go?
* What helped you, what hindered you?
* Were your goals too high or too low?
* Do you feel, health-wise, like you expected to?
* Did you reach your goal?

If you reached your targeted number of points, treat yourself. You earned it! If you did not reach your goal, do not reward yourself! Simply revise your target and start over again.

Continue this exercise weekly for at least four weeks or longer until you are satisfied that the energy and satisfaction resulting from your "cleaned-up" lifestyle has helped you develop new habits which will continue on their own momentum.

61 ONE-A-DAY PLAN

This simple process helps participants formulate a 30-day plan for reaching specific wellness goals.

GOALS

1) To identify specific goals to be pursued and rewarded in the month ahead.

2) To review and reinforce the concepts presented during the learning experience.

GROUP SIZE

Unlimited; works well with individuals, too.

TIME FRAME

20-30 minutes

MATERIALS NEEDED

"One-a-day Planning Calendars" for everyone; blank paper; blackboard or newsprint easel.

PROCESS

Note: This exercise works best when each participant has kept a running list of his dreams, wishes, resolutions and wellness goals throughout the learning experience. (Exercise 48, THE WISH LIST, p 53, would be excellent preparation.)

1) The trainer briefly summarizes the session/course content, inviting participants to mentally review the issues that have been raised for them and the resolutions for change they have made.

2) Participants are instructed to make a list of all the self-care goals they have considered. The trainer encourages people to break large goals into smaller behavioral steps and attitudinal changes.

   Note: The trainer may ask people to share some of their goals with the group at large. This will stimulate participants to consider changes that had not occurred to them and gives the trainer an opportunity to demonstrate how to break large goals into small steps.

3) The trainer offers a few brief comments about motivation, noting that inertia is a powerful force. For most people, making even small changes is a difficult process. The trainer outlines three secrets for success.

- Set challenging yet achievable goals.
- Take one small step at a time.
- Reward yourself for every step as soon as possible, and keep doing so until the change becomes a habit!

4) The trainer draws attention to the reward side of the planning equation, asking people to think about the treats they could give themselves for accomplishing a self-care goal. The group brainstorms an extensive list of rewards that could be used to reinforce the change process. The trainer writes all ideas on the blackboard or newsprint.

Note: If the group gets stuck generating ideas, or if the list lacks diversity, the trainer may need to prompt the group by soliciting suggestions for rewards that are free, or that involve another person, or take less than a minute, or are mental or spiritual, rather than physical -- or any other creative options.

5) The trainer distributes the "One-a-day Plan Calendars" to participants, asking them to fill in the dates for 30 days, starting with today.

Participants are invited to make their own personal 30-day plans by deciding on a wellness goal for each day, and writing it on the calendar. The goal could be the same for every day (eg, smoke no cigarettes, 1500 calories or less, etc), or varied for every day (eg, aerobic exercise 3 times per week, more complicated goals on weekends, increase or decrease during the month, etc).

Using the list of rewards generated in Step 4, participants then choose a treat for each that they can use to reward themselves for accomplishing their day's goal. Again, the reward could be the same every day or could vary with the goal or day of the week. Rewards that can be given and appreciated right away are most effective. It's also better if the reward itself is healthy!

6) When people have finished their planning calendars, the trainer invites anyone who wishes to tell the group about the changes they are planning. The group can show its support with applause, cheers, etc.

ONE-A-DAY PLANNING CALENDAR

SUNDAY	MONDAY	TUESDAY	WEDNESDAY	THURSDAY	FRIDAY	SATURDAY
Goal: Reward:	Goal: Reward:	Goal: Reward:	Goal: Reward:	Goal: Reward:	Goal: Reward:	Goal: Reward:
Goal: Reward:	Goal: Reward:	Goal: Reward:	Goal: Reward:	Goal: Reward:	Goal: Reward:	Goal: Reward:
Goal: Reward:	Goal: Reward:	Goal: Reward:	Goal: Reward:	Goal: Reward:	Goal: Reward:	Goal: Reward:
Goal: Reward:	Goal: Reward:	Goal: Reward:	Goal: Reward:	Goal: Reward:	Goal: Reward:	Goal: Reward:
Goal: Reward:	Goal: Reward:	Goal: Reward:	Goal: Reward:	Goal: Reward:	Goal: Reward:	Goal: Reward:

62 VITAL SIGNS

In this powerful closing exercise, participants affirm directly the signs of vitality which they have seen and appreciated in each of the other members of their small discussion group.

GOALS

1) To provide for each participant the heart-warming, health-giving experience of being affirmed by others.

2) To demonstrate the power of affirmation in human relationships.

3) To provide closure for discussion group members, helping them to bid each other good-bye at the end of the workshop.

GROUP SIZE

Any size group is appropriate.

TIME FRAME

10-15 minutes

MATERIALS NEEDED

A copy of the "Vital Signs" worksheet or a blank piece of paper for each participant.

PROCESS

1) Participants sit with members of their small discussion group (4-6 persons) with whom they have had previous interaction during the workshop.

   Note: With intact staff sessions in which participants already know each other, prior interaction in the small groups during the workshop itself is helpful, but not essential.

2) The trainer asks each participant to reflect individually in writing on the following questions:

   - ☐ Right now one sign of vitality I recognize in myself is ______________________.
   - ☐ I affirm that quality in myself by ______________.
   - ☐ I could celebrate it even more actively by ______ ___________________________.

3) The trainer asks participants to list the names of each person in their discussion group, then to write down next to each name a sign of life and vitality they have seen and appreciated in that person. Participants are to keep these compliments to themselves for the moment.

4) The trainer asks the group to give feedback to each other in the following structured manner. One person will be put in the spotlight for 90 seconds. During that 90 seconds each group member will tell the spotlighted person directly what sign of vitality he has recognized and appreciated in her.

   The trainer should set the structure for this feedback by instructing the receiver to be quiet and listen -- to resist the temptation to laugh with embarrassment or make a remark that wipes out the affirmation. If the receiver says anything it should be, "Thank you."

   The person giving feedback should look and speak directly to the receiver. Participants should not talk in generalities (eg, "Hey, what I really like about John over there is that he seems to be kind of funny sometimes"). Rather, the sharer should look directly at the person and use specifics (eg, "John, I appreciate your fine sense of humor. It brightens me up, too!").

   In the 90 seconds allotted, each participant should share his comment of appreciation with the spotlighted person.

   The trainer should keep strict time, and after 90 seconds ask the group to rotate the spotlight one person to the right.

   The trainer begins by giving each group 10 seconds to decide who will be spotlighted first, then announces the beginning of the first 90-second round of affirmation.

   Note: If the discussion groups consist of unequal numbers of people, as is often the case, the trainer will need to allow an extra round or two to enable every group to complete the cycle and ensure that each person receives the gift of affirmation. Suggest that groups already finished with the process either share some of their feelings and reactions to the exercise, or in some way begin to say good-bye to each other.

5) At the conclusion of the exercise the trainer asks for observations and reflections on the experience, and

comments that the energy level in the room seems much higher than 10 minutes before.

The trainer should also comment on the power of affirmation in all human relationships and encourage participants to develop the habit of regularly offering direct affirmation to others.

6) The trainer claims her 90 seconds pointing out that instructors also need the re-energizing vitality of affirmation. She asks the group to describe her signs of vitality which they recognized and appreciated during the workshop.

Note: If this is embarrassing for you and feels awkward, remember you need warm fuzzies as much as anyone else -- especially at the end of a draining workshop. Compliments improve your energy and health too! Risk it. Do yourself the favor! And model the behavior.

The second result of requesting open positive feedback for yourself will be that the final 90 seconds of the workshop will be filled with positive comments on the experience. Hearing the enthusiastic comments of other participants will create a warm memory of the workshop in the minds of all participants.

When your 90 seconds are up, say "thank you" and bid the group good-bye.

VARIATIONS

- This exercise is designed to be used at the end of a workshop. However, with slight modifications it could fit very nicely at any point in the training design -- especially when the relational aspect of wellness is the subject under consideration.

TRAINER'S NOTES

RECOGNIZING AND AFFIRMING MY VITAL SIGNS

Right now one sign of life I recognize in myself is:

I affirm that quality by:

I could celebrate it more actively by:

The vital signs others see in me:

People In My Group	What I Most Appreciated About This Person

GROUP ENERGIZERS

63 BODY SCANNING

This self-awareness interlude teaches participants a technique for attending to tension spots in the body.

GOALS

1) To heighten awareness of physical tension spots in the body.

2) To practice a simple technique for releasing accumulated tension.

GROUP SIZE

Unlimited

TIME FRAME

2-3 minutes

PROCESS

1) The trainer describes the goals of body scanning to participants.

2) Participants settle back into a comfortable position (seated or lying on the floor), with legs uncrossed and arms resting comfortably at their sides.

3) The trainer asks people to close their eyes and take five deep breaths. After allowing at least one minute for participants to quiet themselves and settle in, the trainer slowly directs the group through the body scanning, giving instructions similar to these:

   - I'm going to take you on an imaginary trip through your body. On this journey through your own insides you will search for tension. Please make careful note of any tension you detect and its specific location.

   - When you discover a tense area you may want to exaggerate it slightly so you can become even more aware of the tension. Say to yourself, "I'm tensing my neck muscles" . . . "I'm tightening my back" . . . "I'm holding my shoulders" . . . "I'm aching my stomach" . . . "I'm hurting myself" . . . Again, notice the tension you're holding and then let go, allowing the tension to drain away.

- Take your time as you focus on each body part. Periodically ask yourself, "Where am I tense?"

- Please now follow me through your body in search of lurking tension. Begin by focusing your attention on your toes . . . simply notice them and how they feel . . . move slowly up your body . . . move your attention to your feet . . . heels . . . ankles . . . shins . . . calves . . . knees . . . thighs . . . buttocks . . . hips . . . genital area . . . abdomen . . . stomach . . . chest . . . back . . . shoulders . . . neck . . . head . . . face . . . forehead . . . arms . . . elbows . . . forearms . . . wrists . . . hands . . . fingertips.

- Please prepare yourself to come back into this room. But before you return, quickly scan your body once more and recall exactly where and in what form you found tension.

4) The trainer gently calls participants' attention back to the group and invites them to share any discoveries they made on their body scanning trip.

TRAINER'S NOTES

Submitted by Mary O'Brien Sippel

64 CHEERS!

Small groups compete in a contest for the most creative wellness cheer.

GOALS

1) To reinforce wellness concepts.

2) To stimulate camaraderie, creativity and humor.

GROUP SIZE

Unlimited

TIME FRAME

10-15 minutes, more time with larger groups.

PROCESS

1) The trainer divides participants into groups of 5-8 persons.

   Note: If the group is small, groups of 3 will work fine.

2) Participants are instructed to recall cheers they used in school for pep rallies and games (eg, "2-4-6-8, who do we appreciate?"; "Give me an "O", give me an "H", "give me an "I", give me an "O", etc). Each group should choose a cheer of their own and modify it to fit some concept of wellness covered during the course (eg, intimacy, eating style, spiritual centering, aerobic exercise). Groups are allowed 5 minutes to create a cheer and practice it.

3) The trainer gathers the large group together and asks all people born in July to "volunteer" as "judges".

4) Each small group presents their cheer to the group at large. (Loudly! Enthusiastically, like cheer leaders! Makeshift wellness pompoms are appropriate!)

5) The judges deliberate and select their favorite. The winning group teaches their cheer to the entire group.

6) Periodically during the remainder of the course, when the group needs re-energizing, the trainer (or any one else) can yell out "CHEERS" -- and the whole group stands up and performs the winning cheer they have learned.

65 EXERCISES FOR THE SEDENTARY

This energizer provides a series of stretches that can be done while seated.

GOALS

1) To help participants relax.

2) To offer participants options for stretching and relaxation they can utilize during long periods of enforced sitting.

GROUP SIZE

Unlimited

TIME FRAME

3-5 minutes

PROCESS

1) The trainer comments on the myth that people who "sit" all day are "relaxed" and "comfortable". Sedentary jobs are stressful on the body! Muscles thrive on being stretched and used -- long periods of sitting in the same position lead to tight muscles.

2) The trainer leads the group through a series of revitalizing stretches that people can do while remaining seated. He reminds the group, with appropriate humor, that these exercises can really be done anywhere -- in the car, at your desk, in the powder room, on an elevator (full or empty!), at the movies, in an airplane, at the symphony, in this session!

   Note: The trainer should sit down, too, and demonstrate each stretch as he describes it to the group.

   - Rotate both feet and ankles in full circles, slowly. (Repeat 3 times)

   - Lift one knee and gently pull it to the chest -- hold for 20 seconds. Then lift alternate leg.

   - Simulate the rowing motion by reaching forward and pulling back. (Repeat 10-20 times)

- Lift one arm, apple-picking style, above the head and extend gently for 10 seconds. Then lift the other arm. (Repeat 2 times)

- Rotate hands and wrists gently and slowly in full circles. (Repeat 3 times)

- Turn head slowly 1/4 turn to the right -- hold for 10 seconds. (Don't strain!) Turn head 1/4 turn to the left, again holding for 10 seconds. (Repeat)

- Tighten buttocks to raise self 2-3 inches. (Repeat 5-10 times)

- Lift both arms over head. Clasp hands and gently lean from side to side.

- Place hands in lap, relax and take three deep breaths.

TRAINER'S NOTES

66 FINGERTIP FACE MASSAGE

Everyone experiences the revitalizing power of touch in this gentle self-care break.

GOALS

1) To provide relaxation and revitalization.

2) To practice a simple self-care technique.

GROUP SIZE

Unlimited

TIME FRAME

10-15 minutes

MATERIALS NEEDED

Relaxing background music if desired (eg, Halpern Sounds, Pachelbel's "Canon in D", sounds of the ocean, mellow guitar or flute music).

PROCESS

1) The trainer invites participants to join in a special treat -- a nurturing self-care technique that can be used whenever relaxation, refreshment or revitalization is needed.

2) The trainer begins the music and directs people to lean back, relax and join her in a gentle face massage, as she reads the "Fingertip Face Massage" script.

Note: The ellipses (....) in the script indicate pauses. The trainer may want to practice the exercise before using it to experiment with the timing and pacing. As written, the routine should ideally take about 9 minutes.

3) After a moment or two of "re-entry silence" following the massage, the trainer solicits comments and reactions from the group, asking questions like:

- What was your favorite part of the massage?
- What felt best?
- What was most fun?
- What was most energizing? relaxing?
- When could you particularly use this technique?

ERTIP FACE MASSAGE SCRIPT

e special to yourself . . . to give yourself . . . a nurturing touch . . . a chance for you fortable . . . relaxed . . . and revitalized nts. . .

to do is to get into as relaxed a position as sitting . . . If you're wearing glasses . . . you may ake off your glasses right now. . .

I'd like you to begin by rubbing your hands together . . . Get your hands just as warm as you can . . . and feel the energy in your hands . . . Continue to rub your hands together . . . and when they become all nice and warm . . . and are feeling good . . . I'd like you to close your eyes . . . and to place your hands on your face.

You may find yourself covering your eyes to block out the light . . . Do whatever is comfortable for you . . . and simply hold the palms of your hands on your face for awhile. . . Feel their warmth on your face . . . and feel those sensations of tenderness that come with holding your face . . .

And now with your fingers begin to gently massage your face . . . Move your fingers gently and comfortably across your forehead . . . allowing your fingers to relax the lines in your forehead . . . and to soothe them . . . Give your forehead the kind of stroking and attention it would like . . .

That may be a gentle touch . . . a soft touch . . . or it may be a harder touch . . . one with more pressure . . . Whatever motion or touch you choose . . . enjoy the activity . . . and give yourself a chance to allow your fingers to relax . . . and comfort your forehead . . .

And now . . . move down slowly over the other areas of your face . . . gently massaging and carassing . . . the area of your eyes . . . Feel your hands and fingers over your eyes . . . and now your cheeks . . . and your nose . . .

Pay attention to what your face may be saying to you . . . Pay attention to what it needs and wants from you . . . Listen to what feels good . . . and enjoy that . . . And then move on to other parts of your face . . .

Continue moving down your face. . . and across your lips . . . and chin . . . and jaw . . . Feel your fingertips and your hands . . . as they massage the lower part of your face . . . And feel your breath on your hands . . . when your hands move across your mouth . . . And enjoy the sensations you have . . . with the warmth of your breath . . . and the warmth of your touch . .

Now that your face has become more relaxed . . . and comfortable . . . and you've given yourself a chance to be as tender with your face as you can . . . I'd like you to experiment with a new way of touching your face . . .

This time . . . use your fingertips to stimulate your face . . . by tapping it . . . gently . . . across your forehead . . .across your temples . . . and cheeks . . . and over your nose . . . Feel the energy that comes as you tap . . . Feel your fingertips dance on your face . . . enjoy that stimulation . . .

And then let your fingertips dance on your head . . . vigorously or slowly . . . whatever comes naturally to you . . . As your fingers dance . . . imagine that you're giving your face and your head new life . . . you're giving it new stimulation . . . And enjoy that feeling of stimulation . . . enjoy the new life.

As you're doing this . . . allow your eyes to begin to feel a glow . . . to feel a kind of waking up and sparkle . . . Feel that sense of sparkle and vitality all throughout your face . . . In your eyes . . . on your cheeks . . . even in your nose . . . your lips . . . and your mouth . . .

Give yourself pleasant, warm thoughts . . . joyful thoughts . . . And take a deep breath . . . as you feel yourself once again . . . through your breathing . . .

Now . . . place your hands on your face . . . as you say good-bye . . . for now . . . Allow your face to say thank you . . . to your hands . . . for giving it this special care and attention . . .

You've filled yourself now . . . with something that you may need . . . And this is something you can do for yourself anytime of the day . . . Whenever your face . . . your body . . . your mind . . . or your spirit . . . need some nuturing . . . some new stimulation. . .

Submitted by Mary O'Brien Sippel

67 GOOD MORNING WORLD

This sequence of gentle yoga stretches and rhythmic breathing is guaranteed to energize the group.

GOALS

1) To get centered and activate mind/body energy.

2) To increase oxygen supply and release muscle tension.

GROUP SIZE

Unlimited, as long as there is space for everyone to stretch out; excellent solitary experience as well.

TIME FRAME

3-5 minutes, may be repeated several times

MATERIALS NEEDED

Tape recorder or record player to play soft, flowing, relaxing music, such as Pachelbel's "Canon in D"; Steven Halpern's "Dawn"; flute, harp or guitar music without a distinct beat.

PROCESS

1) The trainer gives the instructions and demonstrates the "Good Morning World" breathing/stretch routine as outlined below, paying particular attention to coordinating the breathing with the movement.

   Note: The trainer may want to teach this sequence in three 8-step segments ("Salute", "The Pump" and "Airplane"), allowing the group to practice each segment separately before trying the whole routine. Remind participants to listen to their bodies and stretch <u>gently</u>. This is not a contest!

2) Participants follow along as the trainer goes through the steps again. Once everyone has learned the sequence, participants are encouraged to continue the stretch for several minutes, moving at their individual pace and in rhythm with their breathing.

Submitted by Martha Belknap

GOOD MORNING WORLD STRETCHES

Salute

	BREATHE	MOVEMENT
#1	IN	Stand with arms at side (this is "center")
#2	OUT	Palms together in front of chest, elbows bent (prayer pose)
#3	IN	Link thumbs, raise arms above head, arch back
#4	OUT	Thumbs linked, bend forward at waist, reach toward floor
#5	IN	Stand, repeating #3 (arms above head, arch back)
#6	OUT	Repeat #2 (prayer pose)
#7	IN	Return to "center" (rest, arms at sides)
#8	OUT	Rest

The Pump

	BREATHE	MOVEMENT
#1	IN	Stand with hands clasped behind seat ("center")
#2	OUT	Arch back, hands clasped stretch toward floor
#3	IN	Return to "center" (hands at seat)
#4	OUT	Bend over at waist, stretching arms in back up toward ceiling, hands still clasped
#5	IN	Stand, repeating #2 (arch back, reach to floor)
#6	OUT	Return to "center" (hands at seat)
#7	IN	Rest with arms at sides
#8	OUT	Rest

Airplane

	BREATHE	MOVEMENT
#1	IN	Stand and raise arms to sides with right palm up and left palm down ("center")
#2	OUT	Bend to the left keeping arms outstretched
#3	IN	Return to "center" and reverse palms, left palm up, right palm down
#4	OUT	Bend to the right, keeping arms outstretched
#5	IN	Return to "center" (arms out)
#6	OUT	Lower arms to sides
#7	IN	Rest with arms at sides
#8	Out	Rest

68 I'M DEPRESSED!

This humorous energizer demonstrates the mind-body connection and the absurdity of incongruent feelings and posture.

GOALS

1) To illustrate the relationship between feelings and non-verbal expression.

2) To discharge energy.

GROUP SIZE

Unlimited

TIME FRAME

2-5 minutes

PROCESS

1) The trainer asks the group to stand up and directs everyone, at the count of three, to make their own verbal and non-verbal personal gesture of triumph, complete with sound effects (eg, jump and shout "hurrah!"; "high fives"; thumbs up; "sack" dance, etc).

   When the trainer counts to three, participants celebrate their triumphs. The trainer cheers them on, then asks the group to try it again with a little more noise and enthusiasm.

2) The trainer invites the group to try an experiment. This time around, participants are to make the same triumphant gesture, but instead of shouting exultations, they are to shout, "I'm depressed!"

3) The trainer solicits observations and reflections from the group. Most groups comment on one or more of the following points:

   * It's hard to feel depressed when your body is energized.
   * The energy in the room goes up with the noise level.
   * We don't often let ourselves be so enthusiastic.
   * Enthusiasm is contagious.
   * If you're depressed, get moving and make noise!

VARIATIONS

- After Step 2 or 3, the group could divide into dyads and try another experiment in congruence. This time the trainer asks people to make a personal gesture of defeat or depression, allowing all parts of the body to sag, slump and droop. Pay special attention to facial gestures of discouragement. While maintaining this depressed posture, participants are directed to describe to their partner how great they are feeling, using whatever positive and enthusiastic expressions they can think of.

  The trainer solicits comments from the group on this incongruity experiment and invites participants to compare the two experiences.

TRAINER'S NOTES

We learned this technique from Joel Goodman.

69 TAKE A DEEP BREATH

This deceptively simple exercise teaches a five minute relaxation routine that everyone knows and anyone can use.

GOALS

1) To reduce body tension

GROUP SIZE

Unlimited

TIME FRAME

10 minutes

PROCESS

1) The trainer introduces the exercise, saying that many people complain they don't know how to relax, or can't afford to "waste" time relaxing.

   Participants are invited to try a five minute experiment using a relaxation technique anyone can use -- anytime, anywhere.

2) The trainer guides the deep breathing exercise using instructions similar to the script below.

   Note: The best posture for deep breathing is to lie down on a firm surface with knees flexed, feet flat and slightly apart. If the meeting room furnishings or mood of the group preclude this pose, participants can sit comfortably in their chairs, with feet flat and arms supported as much as possible. Backs should be straight, but not rigid.

TAKE A DEEP BREATH

First, I'd like you to close your eyes and get as comfortable as possible . . .
Put one of your hands flat on your chest, and one hand on your abdomen between your navel and your breastbone. Take a deep breath, noticing the movement of your hands as you inhale and exhale.

This time I'd like you to breathe in slowly and deeply through your nose, bringing your breath all the way down into your belly so that it pushes up your hand as much as feels comfortable. Your chest should move only slightly and only as your belly rises.

Continue this slow deep breathing in through your nose and down into your belly, then gently letting your breath go out again at a pace that's comfortable for you . . .

Note: The trainer should pause here for a minute or so, allowing everyone to find a comfortable rhythm. If anyone seems to be having trouble, repeat the last paragraph once or twice before moving on.

Now I'd like you to smile slightly, relaxing your face muscles, while keeping up your own rhythm of breathing. And on the next breath would you please inhale deeply through your nose as before, and this time exhale through your mouth, making a soft and gentle "wooshing" sound, like wind in the pines or the ocean surf, as you blow out.

Let your mouth, tongue, jaw and throat relax as you continue to take long slow breaths in through your nose, deep into your belly and let them out through your mouth with a soft wooshing sound . . .

Focus on the sound and feeling of your breathing as your belly rises and lowers and you become more and more relaxed.

Note: Pause here for 3-4 minutes. If necessary, repeat the last two phrases once or twice during that time to keep the group inhaling deeply and exhaling noisily.

Compare the tension you feel now with the tension you experienced at the beginning of the exercise, and when you feel ready, open your eyes and bring your attention back to this room.

3) The trainer asks for reactions from the group, and then uses these resources to reinforce the idea that relaxation can be easily integrated into our busy lives if we just stop and breathe.

4) With the following suggestions, the trainer encourages participants to "take a deep breath" more often.

- Practice deep breathing 5 minutes twice a day for a week or two.

- Once the technique is mastered, you can use belly breathing on demand -- standing, sitting, lying down, alone or with others. The key is to focus on the movement of your belly, the feeling of air flowing in and out and the comfortable sense of relaxation that accompanies deep breathing.
- Use your deep breathing whenever you feel yourself getting tense -- it only takes a minute or two to reverse the process.

TRAINER'S NOTES

Submitted by Ruth Setterlund who first learned a technique similar to this from the Relaxation and Stress Reduction Workbook (Richmond CA: New Harbinger, 1981).

70 UP, UP AND AWAY

Through this uplifting exercise, participants learn the value of relaxed breathing.

GOALS

1) To demonstrate proper breathing as a tension-reducing activity.

2) To provide a relaxed interlude to the learning experience.

GROUP SIZE

Unlimited

TIME FRAME

2-5 minutes

PROCESS

1) The trainer introduces the exercise by asking everyone to stand up and immediately sit back down.

2) The trainer comments about the amount of effort some people spend simply lifting themselves out of a chair. He then demonstrates how people usually get up from a chair.

   Note: The trainer should exaggerate the amount of effort needed -- take a deep breath, groan, put both hands on the table and slowly stand up with a great deal of effort. Then plop back into the chair with arms and legs flying.

3) Participants try this exaggerated process for themselves.

4) The trainer invites the participants to experience a less stressful way of getting out of a chair. Using the metaphor of a hot air balloon, the trainer directs people, while remaining seated, to close their eyes and visualize a hot air balloon just about ready to take off. As the balloon is inflated, it slowly ascends . . . as it deflates, the balloon slowly descends to earth.

5) The trainer goes through the imagery process again, asking participants to take a deep breath as they imagine the hot air balloon rising and to exhale slowly as it descends.

6) The participants are asked to use this same image again, but this time to "become the balloon" -- rising from their chairs as they imagine the balloon rising.

   After making sure everyone is sitting up straight, the trainer asks people to inhale deeply and imagine they are balloons rising. As they do this participants are to slowly lift themselves from their seat until standing. They then exhale while standing.

   Next, participants are directed to take another deep breath, and as they slowly let out the air, descend softly back to their seats.

7) The trainer may ask for comments and observations from the group. If no one else mentions it, he should reinforce the importance of both visualization and deep breathing as tension-reducing activities.

TRAINER'S NOTES

Submitted by Randy R Weigel

71 WORKING COFFEE BREAK

This novel approach to a simple time-tested technique teaches valuable self-care lessons while providing a break in the action.

GOALS

1) To revitalize body, mind and spirit.

2) To promote a high level of involvement among participants.

GROUP SIZE

Unlimited, as long as there is ample space

TIME FRAME

Variable, but the trainer needs to set specific time limits and keep to them -- folks like to know their parameters.

MATERIALS NEEDED

A variety of refreshments including something nutritious like fresh fruit, nuts, freshly baked bread, cheese, juice, etc.

PROCESS

Note: This technique works best early in group sessions when many people have not yet become acquainted. Be careful not to overuse this icebreaker. Most folks like to have some "duty-free" coffee breaks!

1) As "break time" approaches, the trainer divides the group into teams of 4 or 5 persons, and assigns each team a leader.

   Note: The trainer can either use the "counting off" procedure to ensure randomness, and assign the leadership role to the person whose birthday is latest in the calendar year, or allow the grouping and leading to emerge voluntarily.

2) The trainer gives the teams a task to be completed during the break time (eg, assign a controversial topic related to wellness and tell the team to return with a consensus opinion; ask teams to come up with a list of issues needing to be dealt with in the time left; challenge teams to devise a self-care plan for the first week of a diet or stop-smoking campaign).

3) Following the break, each team leader gives a very brief report to the entire group. The trainer may also want to point out the self-care strategies she observed the group using during the break (eg, healthy snacks, expression of feelings, laughter, contact with others, etc).

VARIATIONS

- The "Duty-free" Coffee Break

  This highly successful variation demonstrates that the trainer is filled with the milk of human compassion. It works best when previous breaks have all been "working" breaks:

  Just before break time, the trainer announces that this is a "duty-free" coffee break -- no tasks to accomplish. Be prepared for a standing ovation!

TRAINER'S NOTES

Submitted by Thomas G Boman

72 YOU ASKED FOR IT

This simple, high-energy exercise helps people practice asking directly for what they want or need.

GOALS

1) To help participants identify their needs.

2) To allow participants the opportunity to confront the risk and overcome the fear of asking for what they want.

GROUP SIZE

Unlimited

TIME FRAME

4-10 minutes

PROCESS

1) The trainer asks participants individually to identify a variety of wants/needs they are experiencing (eg, "I want to be liked", "I am hungry", "I am discouraged", etc).

2) The trainer encourages participants to list a few ways of satisfying each need ("I could find someone to appreciate me" or "to give me food" or "to encourage me", etc).

3) The trainer instructs participants to stand and mill around the room, moving from person to person, asking directly for something they want. The trainer outlines the following guidelines:

   A) Participants are to be as direct and specific as possible. For example, they might say:

      * "I'd like an apple. Would you give me one?"
      * "I'd like a hug. Can I get one from you?"
      * "I'd like a compliment. Please tell me what you like about me!"

   B) The responder is not required to oblige, but may say whatever seems appropriate. For example,

      * "No, I won't"
      * "Yes, here is one"
      * "Sorry, I don't feel like it right now"

C) Participants make the request and receive the response. Then, after listening in turn to their partner's request, they respond as they choose.

D) Participants are not to stop and discuss their feelings, or the responses they receive. They quickly move from one partner to another, completing as many transactions as possible in the time allotted.

4) The trainer reconvenes the group and asks for observations. The following questions may be helpful:

- ☐ What happened?
- ☐ What feelings did you experience?
- ☐ What responses did you receive?
- ☐ Is it really so frightening to ask?
- ☐ Is it really so devastating to be turned down?
- ☐ Where and how could you use what you just learned in your life? With whom? When? What difference would it make for you?

VARIATIONS

- This energizer provides a perfect opportunity for trying out concepts learned in any exercise where participants have already identified personal needs -- especially interpersonal needs. It would be a good companion to THE MARATHON STRATEGY (Wellness I, p 49) or INTERPERSONAL NEEDS/SATISFACTIONS (Wellness I, p 81).

CONTRIBUTORS

Martha Belknap MA
Educational Consultant
395 Monroe
Denver CO 80206
303/321-0905

Marti is an educational consultant with a speciality in creative relaxation and stress management skills. She has 25 years of teaching experience at all levels. Marti offers relaxation workshops and creativity courses through schools, universities, hospitals and businesses.

Thomas G Boman PhD
Professor, Dept of Professional Education
U of Minnesota-Duluth
Duluth MN 55812
218/726-7157 (campus)
218/724-2317 (home)

Tom is a practicing educator, in-service trainer and program developer. His role as founder of the Society for Orthosynergistic Behavior (the study of the right combination of behaviors to enhance high level well-being) allows him ample opportunity to study the maintaining of professional and personal vitality. PhD in Educational Psychology, MA in Curriculum and Instruction, BS in Chemistry.

Joel Goodman EdD
Director
The Humor Project
110 Spring St
Saratoga Springs NY 12866
518/587-8770

Joel has been an advocate of experiential education since his graduate school days at U Mass during the early '70's. Author of several books ranging from values clarification to magic, Joel helps folks get serious about humor through workshops, speeches and the journal he edits, "Laughing Matters!"

Lois B Hart
Leadership Dynamics
Box 320
Lyons CO 80540
303/823-5146

Author of the excellent process exercise collections, Saying Hello and Saying Goodbye, as well as The Sexes at Work, Lois offers workshops and speeches to all kinds of organizations who are interested in the development of their leaders and employees.

Merrill Kempfert MDiv
Director, Parkside Lodge
Alcoholism Treatment Center
24647 N Highway 21
Mundelein IL 60060
312/634-2020 (office)
312/566-2026 (home)

As a Lutheran pastor and administrator of an alcoholism treatment center, Merrill struggles with leading a balanced life, juggling work, family and outdoor interests.

Sandy Queen
LIFEWORKS
1761D Champlain Dr
Baltimore MD 21207
301/298-4522

The author of Wellness for Children and President of the Organization of Wellness Networks, Sandy maintains a busy practice as an independent health consultant. She is best known in the Washington area for her stress management workshops in business and industry. Sandy was recently appointed to the Maryland State Commission on Physical Fitness.

Keith W Sehnert MD
4210 Fremont Avenue S
Minneapolis MN 55409
612/824-5134

Keith is a family doctor who has become a leader in the medical self-care movement. He spends much energy in print (How to Be Your Own Doctor - Sometimes, Stress/Unstress and Wellcare/Selfcare) and in person urging people to improve their physical, mental and spiritual well-being.

Ruth Setterlund BS RN CNP
Student Health Service
U of Minnesota - Duluth
Duluth MN 55812
218/726-8155 (office)
218/728-4986 (home)

A creative, whole person practitioner, Ruth has been bringing the message of wellness to students at UMD and to health care professionals on campuses throughout the midwest and Latin America. Her sensitivity, vitality and zany humor are a superb model for young and old alike.

Mary O'Brien Sippel RN MS
517 Lincoln Park Dr
Duluth MN 55806
218/723-6130 (office)
218/722-8136 (home)

Mary is still one of Whole Person Associates' most enthusiastic faculty. Now a counselor and faculty member at the College of St Scholastica, Mary continues to inspire others to care for themselves and stay vital. Mary's experience in teaching stress management across the country has enabled her to be her own best caretaker as career woman, wife and mother of two toddlers.

Randy R Weigel
Human Development Specialist
Iowa State University
213 Child Development
Ames IA 50011
515/294-8754 (office)

Through workshops, study guides and media development, Randy specializes in making stress research understandable and usable by lay audiences. His training in human relations and education allows him to tailor programs to the needs of specific audiences. Randy has trained students, faculty, parents, farmers and helping professionals in stress management.

THE EDITORS

All Handbook exercises not specifically documented are the creative efforts of the editors who have been designing, collecting and experimenting with structured processes in their teaching, training and consultation work since the late 1960's.

Nancy Loving Tubesing, EdD, holds a masters degree in group counseling and a doctorate in counselor education. She served as editor of the Society for Wholistic Medicine's monograph series and articulated the principles of whole person health care in the monograph, Philosophical Assumptions. A Faculty Associate and Publications Director at Whole Person Associates, Nancy is currently channeling her creative energies into the development of the Handbook series and the compilation and testing of exercises for future volumes.

Donald A Tubesing, MDiv, PhD, designer of the widely acclaimed STRESS SKILLS seminar and author of Kicking Your Stress Habits, has been a pioneer in the movement to reintegrate the body, mind and spirit in health care delivery. With his background in psychology, theology and education, Don brings the whole person perspective to his consultation in business and industry, government agencies and hundreds of health care and human service systems.

Nancy and Don have collaborated on many writing projects over the years, beginning with a small group college orientation project in 1970 and culminating in the publication of their new self-help book on whole person wellness, The Caring Question (Minneapolis: Augsburg, 1983).

FUTURE CONTRIBUTORS

If you develop an exciting, effective structured exercise you'd like to share with other trainers in the field of stress management or wellness promotion, please send it to us for consideration using the following guidelines:

1) *Your entry should be written in a format similar to those in this Handbook.*

2) *Contributors must either guarantee that the materials they submit are not previously copyrighted or provide a copyright release for inclusion in the Whole Person Handbook series.*

3) *When you have adapted from the work of others, please acknowledge the original source of ideas or activities.*

4) *Include a brief (40 words) creative biography similar to those above.*

All contributors will be acknowledged on receipt. The editors will review each submission and test it with one or more groups before reaching a decision about inclusion. Materials must be received by July 1st to be considered for the next year's Handbook volume. You will be notified by October 1st whether or not your exercise will be included.

WHOLE PERSON PUBLICATIONS

KICKING YOUR STRESS HABITS:
A do-it-yourself guide for coping with stress

by Donald A Tubesing, MDiv, PhD

Striking graphics highlight this unusual "workshop-in-a-book" which actively engages readers in identifying sources of stress and resources for coping. Full of examples, worksheets, checklists, practical ideas and a planning process that really works! Ideal for classroom or group setting. Large format paperback, $10.00

THE CARING QUESTION
You first or me first — choosing a healthy balance

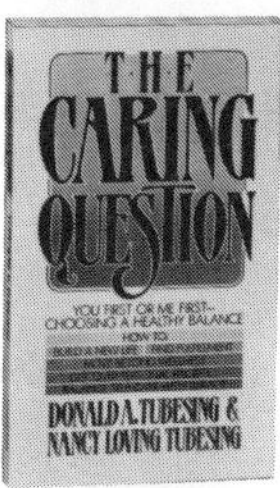

by Donald A Tubesing & Nancy Loving Tubesing

Thought-provoking questions are scattered throughout this startling challenge to the wellness revolution. Filled with wit and wisdom, The Caring Question invites readers to move beyond wellness to a life that balances self-care with caring for others. Paperback, $3.95.

WHOLE PERSON HEALTH CARE: Philosophical Assumptions

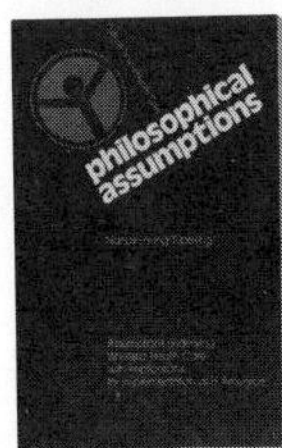

by Nancy Loving Tubesing

This slim volume is packed with insights concerning the nature and form of whole person health care along with snapshots of the theory in practice, challenges to practitioners, and suggestions for research. Paperback, $6.00.

IN OUR OWN HANDS
A woman's book of self-help therapy

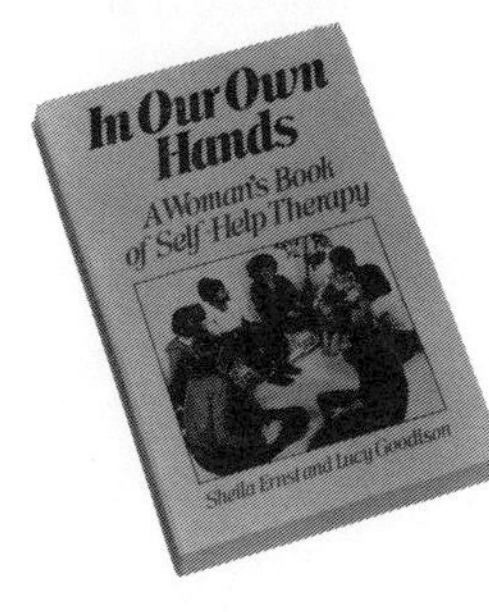

by Sheila Ernst and Lucy Goodison

This practical guidebook for starting a self-help group belongs in the library of every professional who works with groups. Clear, concise descriptions of several theoretical approaches are interspersed with oodles of outstanding exercises that any group could try. Add 143 techniques to your bag of tricks. Paperback, $9.95

TAPE/WORKBOOK TRAINING PACKAGES

STRESS SKILLS: A structured strategy for helping people manage stress more effectively

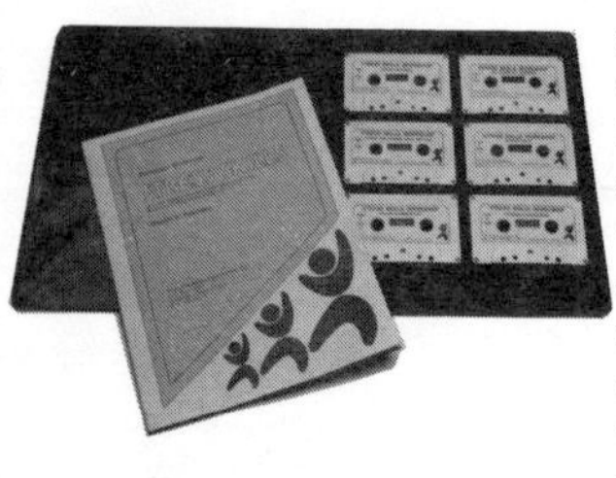

Voice-over narration guides the listener through the celebrated STRESS SKILLS seminar experience captured in these recordings. Concept essays precede each worksheet in the Participant Workbook and highlight topics such as: the nature of stress, taking control of stress, choice and change, whole person stress analysis and 20 stress skills. Perfect for individual or small group study, this resource would be a valuable addition to any staff training library. Six cassettes with companion workbook, $75.00. Workbook only, $6.00.

TUNE IN: Empathy training workshop

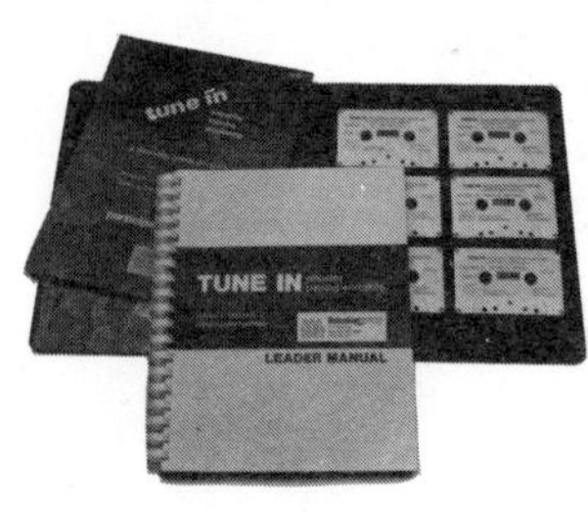

TUNE IN is a carefully developed and extensively tested empathy training workshop you can conduct yourself. The 16 hours of tape-led group experiences help participants develop competency in basic listening and empathy skills. Currently used around the world for inservice training of counselors, teachers, physicians, hospital personnel, volunteers, nurses, clergy, office staff, managers and administrators. Workshop tapes, Leader Manual and Participant Workbook, $75.00. Workbook only, $6.00.

Rx for BURNOUT: Promoting vitality and preventing burnout in the care-giving professions

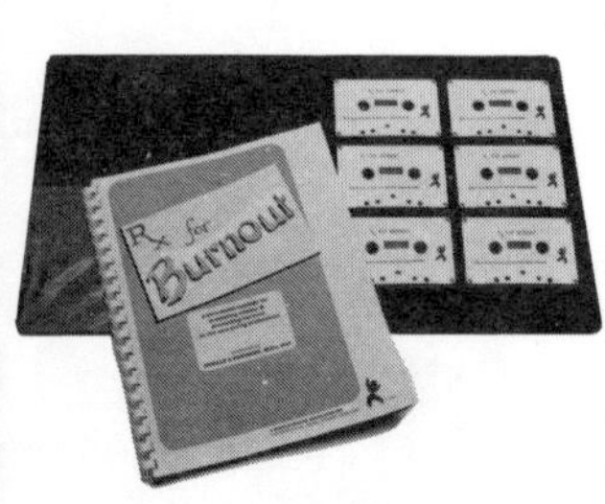

Carefully edited, attractively packaged cassette recordings of a live, Rx for BURNOUT workshop can be used with the accompanying Participant Workbook to create the seminar atmosphere and process. Topics include: symptoms, stages and causes; stress/vitality in the workplace; individual revitalization strategies; interpersonal support networking and planning for renewal. Order this package for conducting your own workshop or to share with friends and colleagues. Tapes and workbook, $75.00. Workbook only, $6.00

UNUSUAL CASSETTE TAPES

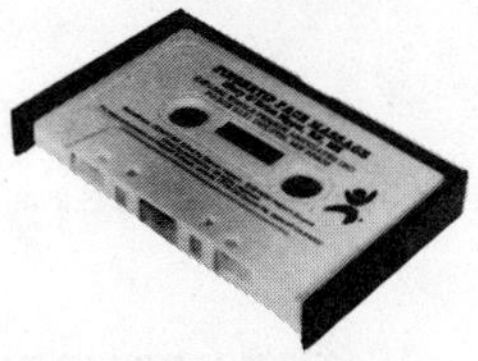

RELAX . . . LET GO . . . RELAX

Music by Steven Halpern provides the calming background for a 30 minute "end of the day" relaxation sequence for shedding tension, and a 20 minute "anytime of the day" revitalization routine. Male and female narration, $9.00.

SPIRITUAL CENTERING: An inward journey of renewal

In this non-judgmental exploration of personal spiritual depths, Don Tubesing guides listeners through a process of quieting and centering that allows each person to discover her own internal wisdom. Useful as a discussion starter or closing motivator. Flip side with Halpern Sounds musical background, $9.00.

FINGERTIP FACE MASSAGE: A gentle self care break

In her warm and gentle manner, Mary O'Brien Sippel guides listeners through a refreshing self-massage process. The 10-minute experience generates a feeling of relaxation, well-being and renewed vitality. Use this tape as an "energy break" during long sessions or to kick off your presentation of self-care options. Flip side with Halpern Sounds musical background, $9.00.

DAYDREAMS: A week's worth of get-aways

You deserve a mini-vacation from stress and strain — use the movie screen in your mind to unstress yourself — take a relaxing guided journey . . . to the seashore . . . for a quiet sail . . . to a sunswept mountain top . . . for a peaceful paddle on a crystal lake . . . to a bubbling hot spring . . . Seven different 5-minute get-aways with soothing environmental and musical backgrounds, $9.00.

BEYOND PEPTALKS AND HANDOUTS

Effective teaching helps people move beyond information to implementation. In this practical presentation, process education expert Dr Don Tubesing shares his philosophy and time-tested techniques for getting participants involved in the learning experience, $9.00.

YOU ALONE CAN BE WELL . . . But you can't be well alone!

In this keynote speech from Wellness Promo VII, Dr Donald Tubesing addresses the issue of wellness from the whole person perspective, asking the question, "What's the point of being well?" Listeners are asked to reflect on the self/other care balance in their lives. A humorous, challenging, positive 90 minutes, $9.00.

THE WHOLE PERSON HANDBOOKS
for trainers, educators and group leaders

STRUCTURED EXERCISES IN STRESS MANAGEMENT

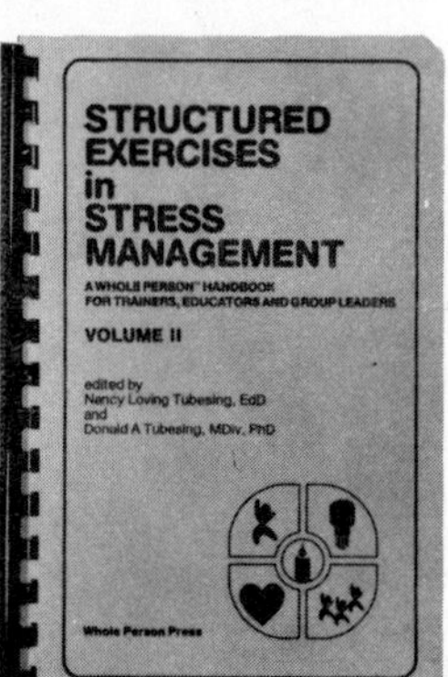

Nancy Loving Tubesing, EdD and
Donald A Tubesing, PhD, Editors

Volume 1 (orange cover) contains 36 ready-to-use teaching designs that involve the participant as a whole person in learning to manage stress more effectively. These exercises help motivate people to identify desired changes, build new coping skills and plan for a healthier lifestyle.

This practical resource includes icebreakers, stress assessments, management strategies, skill builders, action planners and group energizers. Spiral bound, flexible plastic cover, $19.95.

Volume 2 (red cover) and **Volume 3** (yellow cover) each contain 36 all new process teaching ideas in the same easy-to-use format, $19.95 each.

STRUCTURED EXERCISES IN WELLNESS PROMOTION

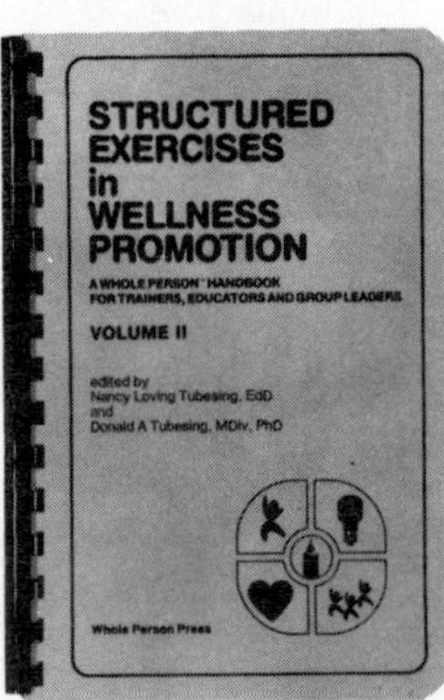

Nancy Loving Tubesing, EdD and
Donald A Tubesing, PhD, Editors

Volume 1 (green cover) includes 36 experiential learning activities that focus on whole person health — body, mind, spirit, emotions, relationships. These exercises encourage people to adopt a wellness-oriented attitude and develop more responsible self-care patterns.

This handy volume contains icebreakers, wellness explorations, self-care strategies, action planners and group energizers. Spiral bound, soft plastic cover, $19.95.

Volume 2 (blue cover) and **Volume 3** (purple cover) each include 36 totally different individual and group exercises that promote wellness, $19.95 each.

THE STRESS KIT

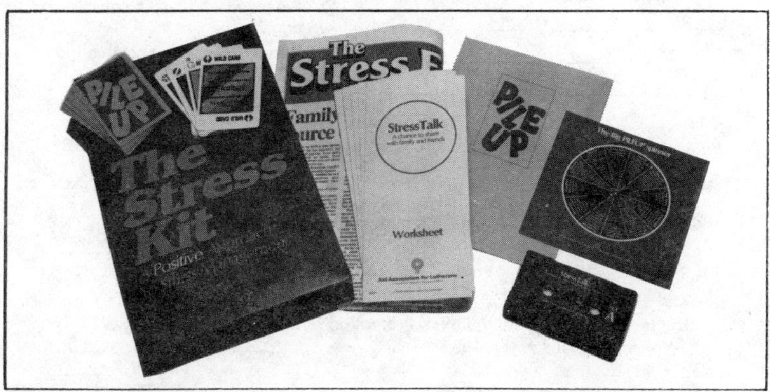

Whole Person Press is proud to announce the latest innovation in stress management resources — a multimedia kit that stresses creative coping. Designed by Whole Person Associates as a health promotion tool for a major insurance company, **The Stress Kit** is now available for your personal or professional use.

The kit includes three educational components — PILEUP (a card game), The Stress Examiner (an unusual newspaper) and Stress Talk/StressRelease (cassette tape programs). This $45.80 value is available packaged together in an attractive bookshelf container for only $29.95. The components may also be purchased separately.

Use one or more of these fun-filled pieces with staff, clients, students, team members, family or friends. You'll understand stress better — and discover positive, effective coping strategies.

PILEUP

A deck of 108 colorful stress and coping cards with instructions for 12 self-discovery games. Card sorts, role plays, assessments, simulations and games graphically demonstrate how stress piles up and how creativity can expand your coping capabilities. Super for families or work teams! $15.95 separately.

The Stress Examiner

This 12-page, 4-color newspaper (USA Today format) is bursting with information and activities for readers of all ages. Test your stress quotient. Play Penny Pileup. Read how celebrities cope. Find out about stress and how to deal with it in every day situations. A book-full of ideas — yet so much more readable! $3.95 separately.

Side A (Stress Talk) of this tape provides a mini-workshop that guides an individual or group in exploring personal stress patterns and management styles. Reproducible worksheets are included for group use. $15.95 separately.

Side B (StressRelease) features a special "radio broadcast" that teaches simple, effective techniques to relieve tension. The program ends with a 15-minute progressive relaxation exercise, complete with mood music. $9.95 separately.

ORDER FORM

Name ______________________

Address ______________________

____

City ______________________

State ______________ Zip ________

Please make checks payable and send to:
Whole Person Associates Inc
PO Box 3151
Duluth MN 55803
218/728-6807

WHOLE PERSON HANDBOOKS for trainers, educators & group leaders

Structured Exercises in Stress Management

☐ Volume 1 (orange cover, 1983)	19.95	____
☐ Volume 2 (red cover, 1984)	19.95	____
☐ Volume 3 (yellow cover, 1986)	19.95	____

Structured Exercises in Wellness Promotion

☐ Volume 1 (green cover, 1983)	19.95	____
☐ Volume 2 (blue cover, 1984)	19.95	____
☐ Volume 3 (purple cover, 1986)	19.95	____

TAPE/WORKBOOK TRAINING PACKAGES

☐ STRESS SKILLS workshop	95.00	____
☐ TUNE IN workshop	95.00	____
☐ Rx for BURNOUT workshop	95.00	____

WORKBOOKS ONLY

☐ STRESS SKILLS Participant Workbook	7.50	____
☐ TUNE IN Participant Workbook	7.50	____
☐ Rx for BURNOUT Participant Workbook	7.50	____

BOOKS

☐ Kicking Your Stress Habits	10.00	____
☐ The Caring Question	3.95	____
☐ Philosophical Assumptions	6.00	____
☐ Wholistic Health	12.95	____
☐ In Our Own Hands	9.95	____

TAPES

☐ Daydreams	9.00	____
☐ Relax . . . Let Go . . . Relax (with Halpern Sounds)	9.00	____
☐ Spiritual Centering	9.00	____
☐ Fingertip Face Massage	9.00	____
☐ You Alone Can Be Well . . . But You Can't Be Well Alone!	9.00	____
☐ Beyond Peptalks and Handouts	9.00	____

☐ **THE STRESS KIT**	29.95	____
☐ Stress Talk (cassette workshop)	15.95	____
☐ Pile Up (educational card game)	15.95	____
☐ StressRelease (radio program cassette)	9.95	____
☐ The Stress Examiner (newspaper)	3.95	____

SUBTOTAL ______
TAX (MN residents 6%) ______
***SHIPPING** ______
GRAND TOTAL ______

☐ My check is enclosed (US funds only)
☐ Please charge my bank card
☐ VISA ☐ Mastercard
Card # ______________________
Expiration date ______________________
Signature ______________________
☐ Bill my institution (PO # ______________)

***Shipping.** We ship UPS in the US. Please include $2.50 for the first item and 50¢ for each additional item. Outside the continental US please add $4.00.